Hot Girl Walk ®

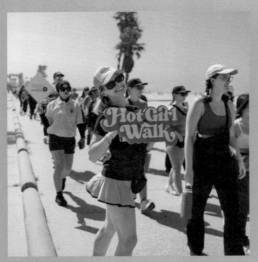
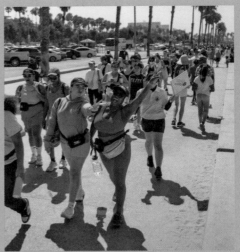
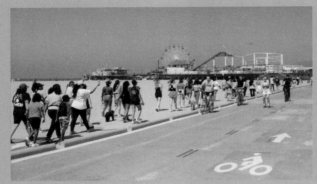
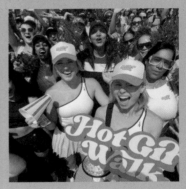
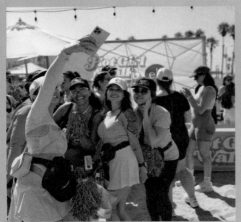
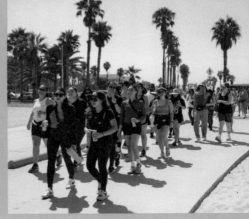

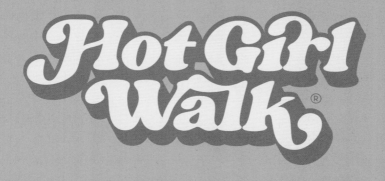

Hot Girl Walk®

FIND HAPPINESS, ACHIEVE YOUR DREAMS, AND CULTIVATE CONFIDENCE

MIA LIND

ROCK
POINT

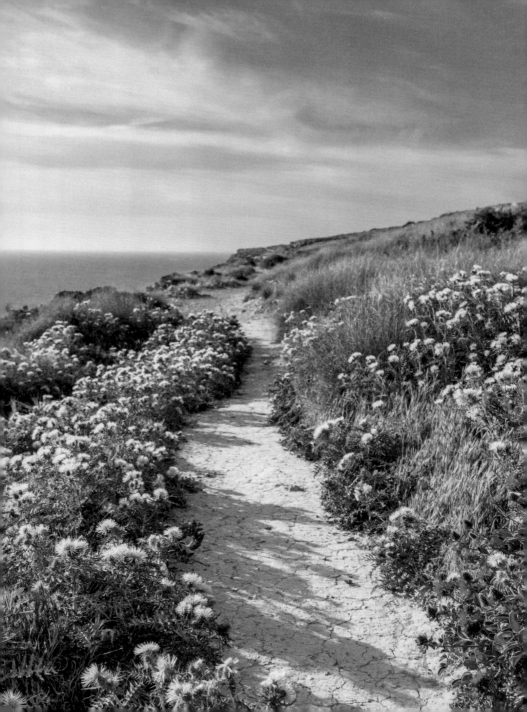

To my younger self

You are stronger and more beautiful than
you give yourself credit for.

Contents

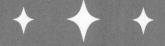

MY JOURNEY & INSPIRATION

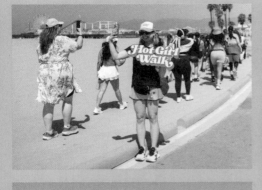
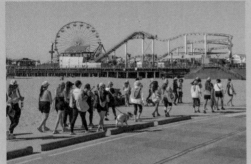
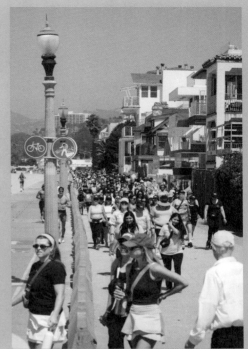
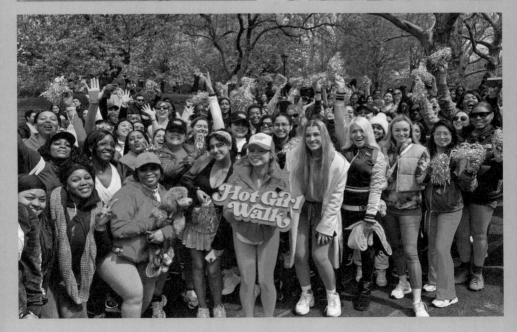

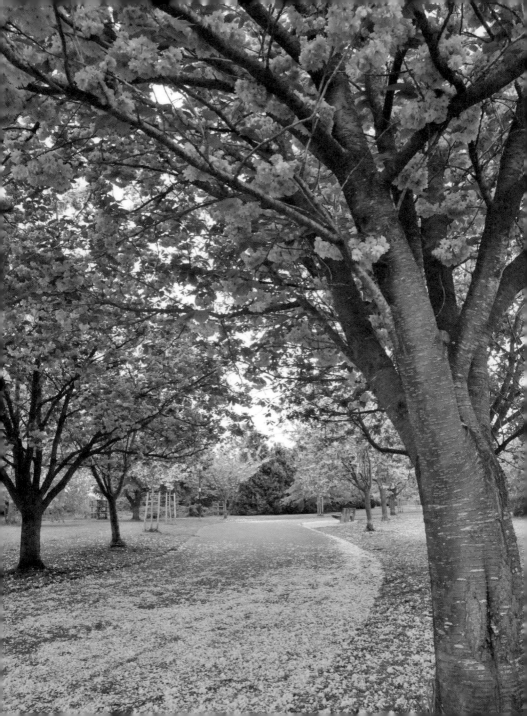

What is a "hot girl"? For me, the idea stems back to social media, specifically Instagram. I was eleven years old when I first heard about Instagram. To preface, I want to note that my bedroom at the time was pink. My mom told me I could paint the walls any color I wanted when we moved from New York to Los Angeles. So, my miniature rebellion was to paint the walls not a light pink but an obnoxious bubblegum pink to match my Pepto-Bismol–colored carpet. My mom warned me to go for the lighter, demure ballerina pink, but I insisted on the bright pink because that's the color that Hannah Montana would have painted her room. Just keep this in the back of your mind; I promise we'll circle back to it.

In that room, I had a playdate with the prettiest girl in school (at least in my eyes). She had long blonde hair and blue almond-shaped eyes and didn't think twice about eating a donut if she wanted one. Let's call her Lisa. Lisa flipped her iPhone toward me and showed me a grid of nine girls. They were all selfies taken from an upward angle in direct sunlight and in one of the small squares was Lisa.

After about five seconds to digest what I was looking at, she asked, "Am I prettier than these girls?"

"Of course!" I quickly answered. "You're, like, sooooo pretty!"

"Thanks."

"What is that?" I asked.

"This is an app called Instagram. You can post photos on your account, kind of like Facebook, but it's only for photos. They do beauty competitions here. You submit your picture to these accounts, and everyone votes on who is the prettiest," Lisa explained.

This was my first introduction to social media: beauty competitions for eleven-year-olds. About two years later, I got an Instagram account. Since that playdate with Lisa, I spent my early adolescence trying to discover what it meant to be a Hot Girl. And it wasn't easy. *Teen Vogue* told me that Hot Girls wear red because it catches a guy's attention. The models in magazines showed me that Hot Girls have six-pack abs. Social media said that Hot Girls definitely *never* use Photoshop and always have a natural thigh gap and perfect skin. Hot Girls, in general, aren't girly either. In *Twilight*, the outwardly girly girl never gets the brooding, good-looking vampire boyfriend. It's the quiet, easily manipulated girl who gets not one but *two* guys fighting over her. However, Hot Girls can be girly when the time is right. On top of all of that, they must effortlessly smell good and wear makeup that doesn't look like they're wearing makeup.

Social media continued to evolve along with my maturity; it became a fixture in our home, school, and Internet culture. Instagram, specifically, was an opportunity to get the best photo of yourself, and you had all the control. Rather than hoping you looked like a model, now there were Instagram models who somehow seemed more realistic than the ones on glossy magazine covers near the checkout counter at the grocery store. Later on, apps that could remove whatever wasn't desirable helped you make yourself look just like those Instagram models—remove a pimple here, whiten your teeth, bring in the sides of your waist, but not too much, because you don't want to be a catfish.

It's no wonder that by the time I was in high school, I spent every day on Instagram studying the bodies of models and following their workout routines to look just like them. Alexis Ren, a famous model, posted her ten-minute ab routine on YouTube, and I used to do it in my bedroom every night and wake up each morning wondering why I still didn't look like her.

This is the culture that social media thrives on. It's an opportunity to portray your life the way you want it to be perceived. And an opportunity to envy the lives of others who appear to be perfect—though we all put the same Sepia or Valencia filters over our images to distract from any imperfections. *Perfection.* This was the focus of my adolescence, though I was fed contrasting messages about what that meant as young women forced themselves to fit into hourglass-shaped holes while also taking aesthetic pictures of eating an entire burger. What I learned was that womanhood is a picture of juxtapositions.

These contradictory messages flooded my head through high school. I never went to prom, nor did I have a date to any high school dance. I surely never had a boyfriend, so I put my energy into my studies because school was the one place I could be perfect. I was addicted to refreshing the site where teachers would upload my grades. That feeling of relief when I saw straight As on my report card was like a hit of adrenaline.

However, my world was shattered when it came to applying to colleges. It turned out that writing an essay about my school career up to that point threw a wrench into my academic confidence—suddenly I hadn't done enough in school. Subsequently, in interviews I'd play down my accomplishments. At my Harvard interview, I was asked if I liked to write, and I said no, even though I was writing short stories in my spare time. The interviewer told me that he didn't think Harvard was right for me. At my Northwestern interview, I was told that I would benefit from attending a party or two because I guess I needed to know how to have a certain kind of fun in order to go there. Rejection after rejection magnified this feeling of "not being enough," and it made me feel like I was far from perfect.

To make matters worse, I was rejected from my dream school: the University of Southern California (USC). The rejections from Harvard and Northwestern were expected, but USC was a shock. My brother was a freshman at USC, and I knew my GPA and test scores matched their criteria. My spirit was completely crushed. But I wasn't going down without a fight. As a Hail Mary,

I submitted an appeal and succeeded: I was accepted to USC for the 2018 spring semester.

While, to me, going to USC was the obvious choice, I had this nagging feeling that I wouldn't fit in—that I didn't belong because of that original rejection. Everyone in my life said I'd be dumb not to accept, so I did. I waited out the fall semester by going to a local community college to get some credits while also working at my high school in the theater department. During the fall, I also auditioned to be on the USC Song Team to start carving my way into the community, even though my gut was telling me I didn't belong. Then I got to the final round of auditions, and I was cut. It felt like a nail in the coffin of my pariah status.

After five long months of watching my peers go to USC football games, attend parties, and join sororities, the spring semester finally rolled around. I said to myself, *If nobody thinks I belong here, I'm going to show them they're all wrong. By the time I graduate, they're going to regret that rejection.*

Once I got on campus, I started off strong: I joined a student organization called Model United Nations and luckily got placed with a roommate I liked. We became fast friends, and freshman year turned out to be a lot of fun while I slowly rebuilt the confidence I had lost. Nobody knew me here, so I didn't have to be a bookworm like I was in high school; I could be the fun, cool girl. This release of my reputation built my confidence a hundredfold.

Eventually, I joined a sorority, and by junior year I was elected chapter president for 2020—a role that freshman-year Mia could have never imagined.

Then it was March 2020, and my life turned upside down. As if I wasn't anxious enough about my duties as president—I felt so much imposter syndrome, second-guessing every decision I made and meeting I gave—now I was faced with a global pandemic. As a young leader, my sorority looked to me with questions that not even the president of the United States could answer:

"How long is this going to last?"

"When will we be back to school?"

"Do I have COVID?"

"When will there be a cure or vaccine?"

The year was tumultuous. I went home to my family, all of whom were going through similar feelings of uncertainty. My dad often attempted to lighten the mood, reminding us of the annoyingly optimistic quote his dad used to say: "Think of it as an adventure." A quote that would show up in the most inconvenient of times but ring true when we all had enough perspective.

My problems paled in comparison to many people around the world, but I couldn't help this feeling of frustration. Usually, I could silence it for a little bit when I doomscrolled on TikTok or binge-watched *Breaking Bad*. But COVID amplified the noise on social media.

"If you're not exercising and trying to lose weight during COVID, you're being lazy."

"Everyone can run a mile!"

"If you're not running during COVID, you're out of shape."

Like many people, I got sucked into peer pressure and tried my hand at running. With my best attempts, I could go half a mile at a twelve-minute pace before feeling like I'd pass out. After a month, I gave up and decided I would never be a Hot Girl.

Near the end of my term as chapter president, in November 2020, I'd had enough of being stuck at home and knew I needed to get out. I craved my running era because at least then I got out of the house—yet I also loathed it. I remembered how much I used to walk when I was on campus, easily hitting 10,000 steps a day. So, while it seemed antiquated and lame, I decided to go for an outdoor walk. My neighborhood was in a 4-mile loop, so, with some quick calculations, I knew I could walk for at least an hour and twenty minutes. But even so, walking wasn't really an exercise . . . I could shop for an hour straight, which is kind of the same thing . . . right?

Except, while walking seemed like a simple concept, I found myself hesitating, wondering, *What happens when I'm alone with my thoughts?* I knew what normally happened: I would overthink everything. All my anxieties started screaming in my head all at once. But in spite of knowing that, I was a senior in college now, about to graduate into the real world and get a real job. And I couldn't repeat the disaster of interviews that I had gone through for college, so I needed to make a change.

On my first walk, I thought about the things I was grateful for. In a class I took during high school, they taught us that the secret to happiness is gratitude practice. With nothing better to do, I finally decided to listen to the professionals. Naturally, I thought about the achievements I had made. I had navigated my sorority through a global pandemic . . . that's pretty badass if you ask me. I was getting *A*s in school while holding an internship the entire time. Though my world seemed to be crumbling around me due to COVID, I was starting to recognize that things weren't so bad.

For the first time in my life, I looked at my accomplishments as if I actually deserved them rather than constantly discrediting myself. Nobody could hear these thoughts going through my head, but I had Britney Spears in my ears and endorphins flowing through my veins to boost my confidence even more. The feeling reminded me of the way my guy friends talked about their achievements (because apparently men never had anyone in their heads telling them their successes weren't enough).

Through that simple gratitude practice, I realized I had achieved so much. I could do anything I set my mind to. Soon, the thoughts asking *what's next*

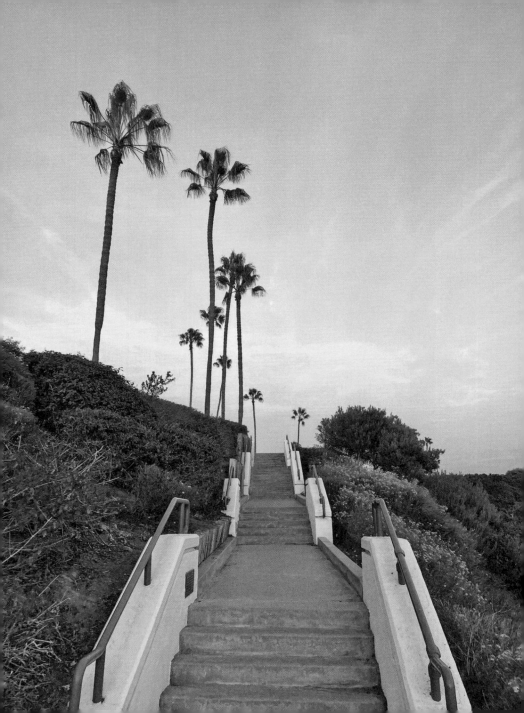

for me? started trickling in. Maybe I'll get a job at a big corporation. I could work up the corporate ladder and become the CEO of a Fortune 500 company. I envisioned myself walking through New York City, heading up to my corner office, or waving to my secretary as I entered my board meeting to discuss our future IPO. Or even walking in a Victoria's Secret Fashion Show, even though I was 5-foot-3-inches (1.6 m) tall and would never be invited. It didn't matter to me; I could be anything I wanted to be. The world finally felt open.

The answer to the question "What is a Hot Girl?" became clear to me: I was already hot. I had spent my adolescence trying to mold myself into somebody I wasn't, and, therefore, I didn't have any confidence. But once I started to stand tall in my own body, suddenly my internal monologue was at peace for the first time in my life. I started to call these walks my Hot Girl Walks.

Opening the voice memos app on my phone, I noted what I focused on during my Hot Girl Walk. When outdoors, there's only one rule, and that's that you can only think about three things: (1) the things you're grateful for, (2) your goals and how you'll achieve them, and of course, (3) how HOT you are.

I did these walks every day for months, had these inner dialogues with myself, and watched my life change before my eyes. I exercised for fun, applied for jobs, and finished my college degree with my best grades yet. I opened up to my sorority sisters about how these walks made me feel, and then they started doing them every day around their respective neighborhoods. One of them, who had gone viral on TikTok for her legendary dances, told me that these walks would also go viral. Everybody agreed and said, "We must tell people what the Hot Girl Walk is!"

In January 2021, I posted the first video, announcing the Hot Girl Walk (HGW) to the world. Within minutes, the video had hundreds of thousands of views on TikTok. The next day, people were taking Hot Girl Walks of their own and soon the video grew to 3 million views, with so many people taking Hot Girl Walks around the world.

I received thousands of messages about how Hot Girl Walks were the reason people got out of bed for the first time in months, how they helped people through quarantine, and so much more. Hot Girl Walks had already helped so many people, so I knew they had the power to help even more. Inspired by my college business classes, I began the early stages of starting a business, and I filed for a trademark.

Meanwhile, after using my Hot Girl Walks to prepare for my job search and many hours of walking, I accepted a job at a big tech company in their sales program. Here, I learned how to cold call and get high-level executives on a meeting with a twenty-two-year-old fresh college graduate. I realized that the younger, less confident version of myself would have shuddered at the thought of calling someone out of the blue, and yet I was making hundreds of these calls daily (and oftentimes getting yelled at and hung up on). Fast forward a bit and I was the top sales representative on my team and quickly promoted to an account executive role where I was closing large-scale, million-dollar deals, learning the true art of sales, and navigating corporate America.

While working full-time, I continued to build Hot Girl Walk as my passion project. If there's one thing I learned as president of my sorority, it was how to build a community, and in my corporate job, I was craving the support of a sisterhood more than ever. The next step for Hot Girl Walk was to become an in-person community event. The first one was attended by 100 people. The next, 200 showed up, and before I knew it, I was flown to New York City to host a Hot Girl Walk with Strava for International Women's Day, where we raised $250,000 for charity, with our virtual challenge including over 220,000 participants from over 190 countries.

After a year and a half of working two full-time jobs, and with help from my mom to grow my business, I quit my corporate job to take Hot Girl Walk worldwide. Today, we have anywhere from 300 to 800 attendees at our events. We have Hot Girl Walk-ed in the cities of LA, Miami, New York, Boston, Las Vegas, and Austin, and have ventured across the ocean to Australia and London.

This book will teach you what Hot Girl Walk can do for you. The most positive thing to come out of Hot Girl Walk is the individual people I've met, including those who tell me how it has changed their lives. This past year, I've met tens of thousands of people, all with unique stories. There are three main themes of the Hot Girl Walk (gratitude, goals, and self-confidence), but this book breaks it down even further to help you achieve your goals and become confident in whatever you choose to do. With exercises to help you get into the habit of self-reflection, you'll find actionable and practical steps, plans, and routines that offer simple and easy ways to conquer everything from everyday challenges to significant fears. If your goal is self-growth of any kind, follow along chapter by chapter and grow into your best self. These are the lessons I've learned from doing my own Hot Girl Walk practice, and the lessons I've learned from others during community Hot Girl Walks.

The world is constantly telling you that you don't have the tools to be your best self, but the purpose of this book is to teach how the power is already inside you. Reclaim the lost art of girlhood: the childlike desire to paint your world bright pink, dress how you want, listen to guilty-pleasure pop music, and take up as much space as you need. You are not made to fit in an Instagram-sized square—the world has enough space. You're already HOT; now let's bring it to the surface. You are a HOT GIRL. It's time to go on your Hot Girl Walk!

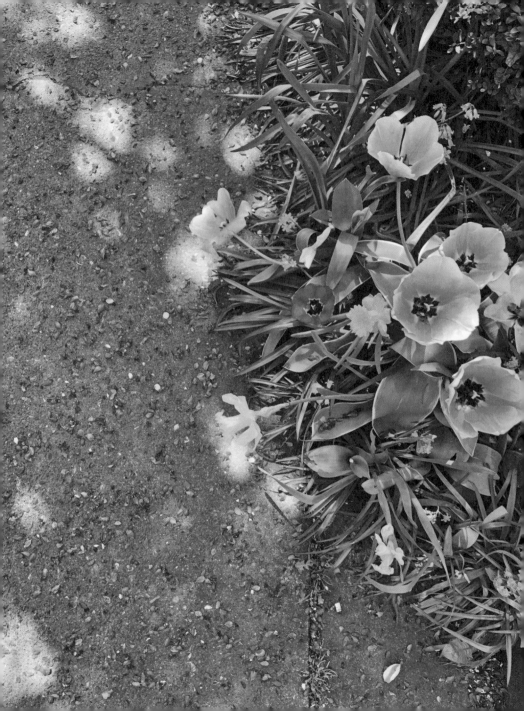

CULTIVATING GRATITUDE

25

THE IMPORTANCE OF Gratitude

27

WHAT IS Gratitude?

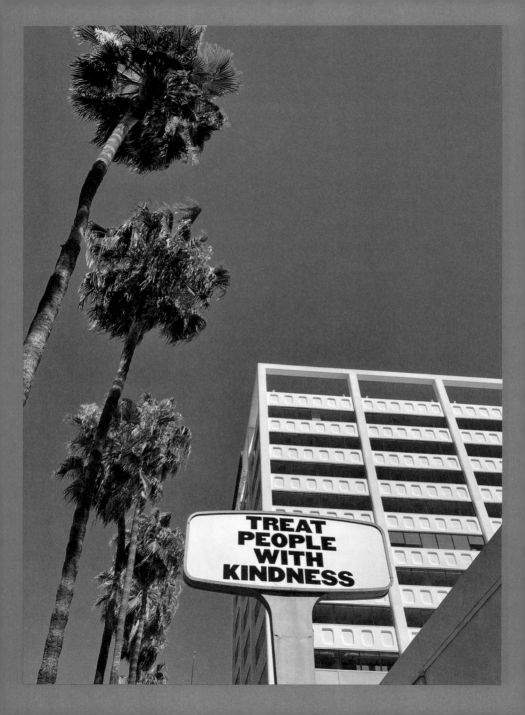

The Importance *of* Gratitude

Before I started Hot Girl Walks, I had a lot of anxiety centered around walking. It sounds silly, but I needed to understand what was holding me back from exercising, and I recognized I had a lot of anxiety associated with being alone with my thoughts—which is exactly what happens when on a walk alone. This mindset was holding me back from reaching my fullest potential. This fear was a microcosm of the anxieties I felt in other areas of my life. I was rarely ever alone with my thoughts; to avoid them, I would doomscroll on TikTok or binge-watch television—even when I was brushing my teeth.

The feeling of anxiety associated with being alone with my thoughts wasn't exclusive to working out or going on a walk. It had been a thread throughout my entire life and was only amplified when I became the president of my sorority in college. I was constantly filled with thoughts of: "What if the worst thing happens? What if people disagree with me? What if I'm not the right person for this?" Constantly calculating every possible consequence of every decision was exhausting and paralyzing. I would stay up late replaying conversations with my friends, wondering if I had said the right thing and worrying that the worst feelings and thoughts I had about myself were true.

Suffice it to say, the overly critical voice in my head (I call her Mean Mia) was not someone I wanted to listen to. I wanted to be able to go on an hour-long walk without a podcast of someone else's thoughts filling my brain simply because I needed to keep my own thoughts quiet.

With Hot Girl Walks, I started on a bigger journey to confront the root of my problem. There's a time and place for forgetting your problems, but this wasn't that time or place. Instead of pairing exercise with my big, scary thoughts, I chose to turn it into a coping mechanism that would help me build the strength I needed to challenge the voice in my head.

So I laced up my sneakers and put on my "pregame" playlist, which included songs I'd play with my girlfriends before going on a fun night out—if I had to listen to someone in my head it may as well be Britney Spears, with her iconic voice, unbridled confidence, and quick, upbeat songs that I could keep a walking pace to.

Forcing myself to ignore Mean Mia, I focused on the things I was grateful for. For as long as I mentally could, I walked and practiced gratitude, and for the first time in my life, I felt happy with where I was. This is the power of gratitude. There are so many ways my life could've turned out, but I was lucky enough to live in a place where I could go on walks year-round and in a time where I could listen to Britney Spears on demand. My family was healthy, and I had friends I trusted and loved spending time with. Turning exercise into a moment of gratitude gave me the chance to settle my mind and build myself up for the next thing life threw my way.

What *Is* Gratitude?

Gratitude practice allows you to get into the right headspace no matter what may be going on in your life. It helps you gain some perspective and recognize what you have to be grateful for rather than fixating on what may be stressing you out right now. It's for this reason that multiple studies have shown a correlation between gratitude and happiness.

According to research by Dr. Sonja Lyubomirsky, 50 percent of your happiness is due to genetics, 10 percent to life circumstances, and 40 percent is based on your actions. Learning this statistic was extremely comforting to me. So often it feels like circumstances are so far out of our control, but this study showed that we *are* in control of our happiness.

Of course, a happy person isn't happy 100 percent of the time, but happiness should exist *despite* life circumstances, not *in spite* of them. For example, being overjoyed with happiness after a breakup would not be genuine happiness, especially if the breakup was challenging. A "happy person" will allow themselves to navigate the roller coaster of emotions and experience happiness when the time is right.

Discovering what happiness means to you as an individual is a big part of the self-exploration journey that Hot Girl Walks can help you uncover. As I was faced with tough challenges, it was difficult for me to

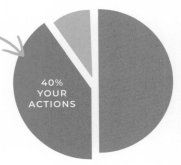

40%
YOUR
ACTIONS

navigate my emotions: to genuinely feel but not let myself fall victim to my circumstances and plunge into a negative spiral. Then I started paying attention to that 40 percent, the portion of happiness that is dependent on my actions. Which leads me back to gratitude.

Now that we know we have some control over our happiness, how do we take action and use gratitude?

If you've genuinely thanked someone for something they did, you know how powerful feelings of gratitude can be. When we take a moment to recognize the numerous things we have to be grateful for, it's somewhat of a "glass half full" feeling. Gratitude is as simple as saying "thank you" for the things that you did not cause. For example: say "thank you" to your body and its ability to get up and walk or to your friend who always answers your phone calls. When you genuinely start thanking the people and things around you for how they contribute to your life, you begin to realize just how much there is to be grateful for.

Additionally, our brains reward us for feelings of gratitude by releasing endorphins (or "feel-good" chemicals). There is evidence that suggests this positive reward system has been supported by evolution. Humans have evolved through history largely because of teamwork. Being able to communicate and work as a team has helped humans accomplish incredible feats and increased their chances of survival. Expressing gratitude to one another is a prosocial behavior that can help support community and, ultimately, growth.

Think about the last time you worked in a team with the same goal—maybe it was a school project or a client presentation at work. Did you receive proper credit from your teammates for the work you put in? If not, you probably felt annoyed or unappreciated and therefore less likely to work as hard the next time. But if you did receive full credit, you probably felt happy and more willing to work again with the person who thanked you for your contribution.

The same goes for the last time you helped someone in need. At a time when you weren't required to help but you did, that person probably gave you their gratitude, which in turn makes you more likely to help someone else again.

Gratitude is a practice that our brain supports by releasing those feel-good chemicals. In other words, gratitude is the biggest life hack to happiness. It's dopamine that comes from recognizing what we already have rather than making us desire what we don't. You have all the tools needed for happiness; you just have to access them.

This is what I came to realize during my Hot Girl Walks. Walking became my time to simply be. My critical inner monologue quieted, and the sense that "everything is going to be okay" made my life so much better.

Gratitude or Candy?

There are many types of dopamine: some require constant upkeep and energy, while others require only a small dose but have a long-lasting effect. Candy, for example, gives you a short boost of dopamine from sugar and carbs. But like most processed foods, it is built to make the first bite the best, while the rest of the experience falls flat. Which makes you reach for another . . . and another, until you have a pile of wrappers on your lap, an ache in your stomach, and maybe some feelings of guilt.

Gratitude, on the other hand, is about eating one piece of candy and savoring every single bite. Eat it mindfully, let yourself enjoy it without guilt, and then you can move on still feeling the effects long after.

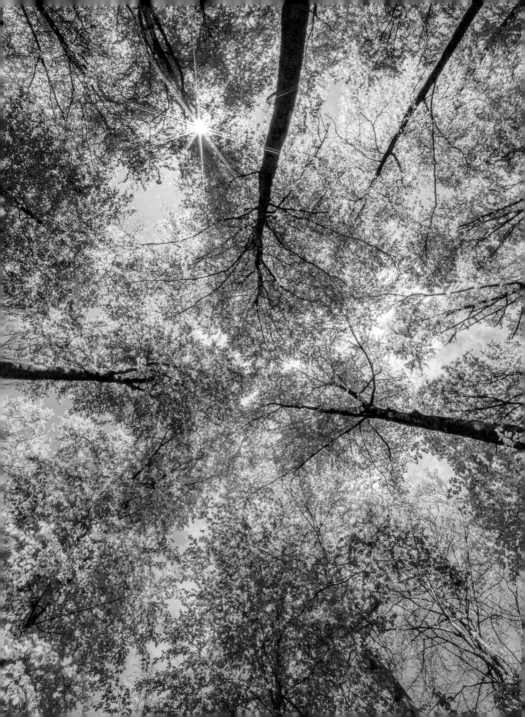

The Tree of Gratitude

To truly practice gratitude, put yourself in a mindset of mindful observation. At the start of the walk set aside whatever may be on your mind and observe what is around you. Look at your surroundings without judgment and try to observe something that you may have never noticed before.

Try this quick exercise to help you foster gratitude daily:

1 Let's check in on your body. Recognize the position you are currently in. Are you holding this book (physical, electronic, or your phone if listening to the audio) with one hand or two? How is your posture? Is your jaw clenched? If so, that's okay. Take a big, deep breath: feel both of your lungs expand and release any tension.

2 If you're holding something, what does it feel like in your hands? If you're not holding something, pick up the closest object to you. Take another deep breath. Feel your chest rise, your ribs expand, and then, as you exhale, feel the air being released from your body.

3 Let's listen to what's going on around you. Is there a fan running? People speaking? A refrigerator humming? Take note of these sounds without judgment. Then take another deep breath and listen to the sound of the air rushing through your nose and out through your mouth.

4 Let's take one final breath. This time recognize what the room smells like. Maybe you smell the pages of a new book, dinner cooking on the stove, or a candle you lit earlier.

Through this exercise, you used three different senses: touch, hearing, and smell. Three things you can be grateful for right now. Once you begin the tree of gratitude, you realize the branches of what you can be grateful for are infinite.

The Miles of Gratitude

Gratitude practice is a *practice* for a reason. It takes trial and error to practice mindfulness and positivity. It may not make much sense the first time—it won't be perfect, but it's not meant to be. If you're new to Hot Girl Walks, I recommend doing this exercise to get used to looking at the world with fresh eyes—with a perspective that isn't clouded by negativity or anxiety about what you may be dealing with.

Mile 1: Start by saying "thank you" to the weather—the warmth of the sun on your skin, the cool breeze brushing your face, or the beauty of a clear sky. We often complain about the weather, but we hardly ever let ourselves feel the beauty of each season. Whether you're feeling hot or cold, appreciate the change of the seasons and how this season is just as fleeting as the next. Enjoy it while you can. Notice the vibrant colors of flowers on your path or the sounds of leaves rustling in the wind— things once easily overlooked when caught up in the chaos of thoughts.

Mile 2: Shift your thoughts toward more personal reflections. Become aware of your body—your legs carrying you forward, your breath steady and strong. Feel the sweat beads on your forehead and recognize your body's instinct to cool you down. Feel a profound sense of appreciation for your health and physical capabilities. It's no small thing; being able to move freely is something many take for granted.

Mile 3: By the time you reach Mile 3, your thoughts may have evolved even further, becoming more introspective and spiritually meaningful. Feel gratitude for the intangibles—your personal growth, the strength you've built from overcoming hardships, and the relationships that have supported you along the way. Reflect on how everything in your life, even the struggles, has contributed to you becoming the person you are today. You may have gone on your Hot Girl Walk to de-stress from your current challenges, but now you recognize how much you've already overcome, and how each obstacle makes you stronger.

While Hot Girl Walks are usually 4-miles long, start here with 3-miles. Allow yourself to recognize what you may not often notice. It seems insignificant to think so small, but as your walks and gratitude practice progress, you will begin to understand how significant a role gratitude can play in your happiness.

In our busy lives, we are often blind to the miracle of our existence. Gratitude practice allows you to shed ideas of success and the pressures of society. At the end of the day, whatever may be stressing you out, realize that things are not so bad after all.

Seek-and-Find

To do a gratitude seek-and-find, as you walk, look around and find as many things as you can to say "thank you" for. If you're struggling, remember that walking itself releases endorphins, helping those positive feelings flood in.

You can also try picking a color during your walk. Whenever you see the color, take a picture of it. You might notice some vibrant orange flowers or a turquoise garage door that happens to match your sneakers. Taking pictures and videos of small moments that you normally wouldn't pay attention to helps you stay grounded and keeps you looking around with fresh eyes and a refreshed mind.

Inspired by
Annabelle's
Story

I learned about the concept and power of gratitude practice when I was in high school. There is something about adolescence that deludes us into thinking that we know more than adults. This was precisely the experience I had. Gratitude practice just seemed lame and like a waste of time. I decided I knew better than the researchers at UC Berkeley and the real secret to happiness was chocolate, watching Bella and Edward fall in love in *Twilight*, and shopping. It took a global pandemic and about four more years of maturing to give gratitude an honest try.

However, as I grew up, my stressors grew as well, and I had no productive coping mechanism to deal with this stress. When I was in college, for example, I'd release stress by getting ice cream with my friends, watching a lot of television, or heading to a frat party. All these things are fine in moderation, but they become cyclical. The more television I watched, the less I'd study for my exams, and the more stressed I'd become; therefore, I'd watch more television and the cycle continues.

My college experience was interrupted by COVID, when some of these mechanisms for dealing with stress were no longer accessible to me. Then, of course, I created Hot Girl Walk, and it became my favorite way to deal with stress. It was also productive because, rather than just being a Band-Aid for my stress, it allowed me to confront it: I'd finish my Hot Girl Walk with a clear mind, and I'd be ready to tackle whatever may have been stressing me out, be it a test, job application, or boy drama.

Since the invention of Hot Girl Walk happened while I was at school, it was so exciting to see that when Hot Girl Walk went viral, it spread like wildfire across college campuses. This attention pushed us to create a program for college students to start Hot Girl Walk chapters on their campuses. Annabelle, a HGW Ambassador from Ohio State University, gives insight into what she loves about Hot Girl Walk as a college student:

> **I love Hot Girl Walk because it helps me mentally and physically. It eases my stress and helps me to relax while also allowing me to feel productive and accomplished. I always feel so much better after my walks. Hot Girl Walk has saved my mental health, helped me think more positively, and kept me motivated and active in college."**

College is the perfect time to learn and develop healthy coping mechanisms. While college can be stressful, it is less stressful than having your first *real* job, being responsible for your taxes and healthcare, and all the other exciting parts of adulthood. Yes, having fun in college is important, but it's also the time to develop tools that you can use moving forward. Remember, it's easier to create new habits than it is to break bad habits.

SETTING & ACHIEVING GOALS

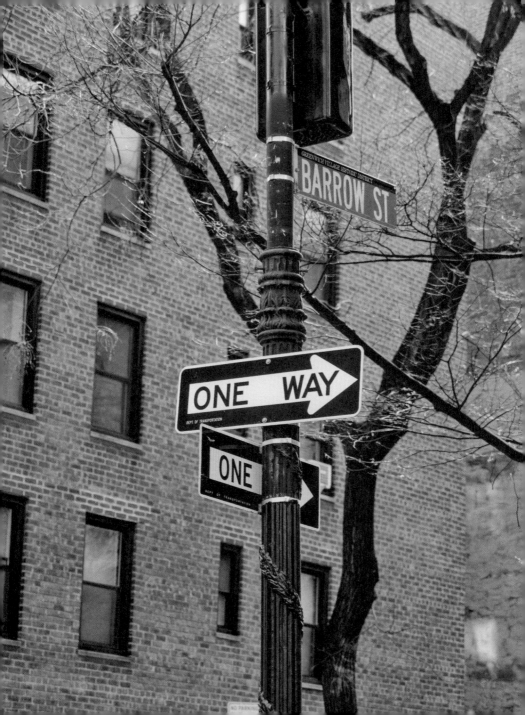

Defining Your Goals

When I got the text asking if I wanted to accept my nomination for chapter president of my college sorority, I felt my stomach drop. At the time, it seemed like that role was too far out of my reach for me to even consider. I called my mom to tell her how ridiculous it was, but she immediately challenged my self-doubt. In fact, she encouraged me to go for it but told me to do one thing before making my decision: go on a walk.

"Just walk around going to your classes today like you're *already* the president," my mom said. "Take note of how it feels and see if it's a position you'd like to have."

Easy enough, I thought. I walked out of my class with my head held high. And with every step the possibility of pursuing this position became more real. I felt so confident and knew I had the power to take up this role. This was about one year before I started my business, but without knowing it, I had taken my very first Hot Girl Walk.

Visualization became my daily practice. When I started going on Hot Girl Walks, I used the time replacing ideations of doom with positive thoughts. There was no limit to who I could be on my Hot Girl Walks because these personas existed in my head. More importantly, I was walking with confidence. I didn't have confidence in my daily life, so I practiced confidence on my Hot Girl Walks. I was giving my brain muscle memory—to view myself in a positive light, for my legs to stride assuredly, and for my body to stand tall.

The way you view yourself holds a lot of power. Many times, I put myself into a "self-fulfilling prophecy" of failure. A self-fulfilling prophecy is a psychological theory where one's negative ideas and thoughts about themselves produce an outcome that fits their expectations. In my case, I would anticipate failure and imagine what would happen if my plans failed, and then they often did. My failure was my own doing. The following exercise, Hot Girl Walk *As If*, has the opposite effect. The idea is to start with the mindset that you can and will succeed. Like when I was visualizing being chapter president, I went about the election process like I had already won. Therefore, I came across as confident and sure of myself, emanating an energy that said: I'd be a good chapter president. By visualizing myself succeeding, I created more positive thoughts in my head, generated confidence to get the job done, and took action to make it happen. Don't walk with self-doubt: walk with no doubt in your abilities.

Hot Girl Walk *As If*

I call this method: Hot Girl Walk *As If*. Meaning, Hot Girl Walk *As If* you already have reached your goals, whatever they may be. This is a scenario-based method where you convince yourself that in any given scenario, you've already walked away with a win. It's about starting with a confident mindset so that you handle the situation with confidence. When practicing this visualization technique on your Hot Girl Walk, imagine you are literally walking a mile in someone else's shoes.

By practicing this method weekly, you can experience:

★ **Positive self-talk.** If you often find your internal monologue filled with criticism, adding positive self-talk can help quiet those voices.

When you're young, you are taught to always say "I can" rather than "I can't," but as you grow into adulthood, that message gets washed away by pressures of success. Let's reinstate positive self-talk to help combat these pressures.

★ **Walking and standing taller.** When we practice confidence, we also need to perform with confidence. Namely, our walk needs to be assured, and our posture should be straightened. When walking toward something difficult, changing the way you physically hold yourself can help a lot when it comes to feeling confident.

★ **Confident decision-making.** Making good decisions each day can be a challenge, and there's no bigger challenge to overcome than the fear of making the wrong choice. You need to trust yourself before you can trust your decisions.

★ **More achievable goals.** A combination of all these things—defined goals, positive feelings about yourself, poise, and consistently making good choices—can result in seeing your goals come together right before your eyes.

If you're going for a job interview, Hot Girl Walk *As If* you already have the job. Imagine what it would feel like to walk into the office after working there for two years. Do you walk nervously and second guess each step? *No.* You're confident in yourself and know that you have the qualifications to get the job done. This is the energy that you need in your interview.

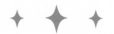

The *Future* Is Yours

You need to be specific about the future version of yourself. The clearer an image of who this person is that you have in your mind, the better you can embody them. It's a chance to get down to the little details, like how they dress and speak, and what they do in the mornings. When you picture the minutiae, it challenges you to think in the mind of your "best self" and know every corner of your best self's brain. This can be a hard thing to do, so to help, I've created the following worksheet.

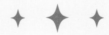

Who Is Your Best Self?

Let your imagination run wild and visualize your most ideal life. Leave being humble at the door and imagine what a day in life would look like if you achieved all your wildest goals—down to eating a healthy breakfast each morning.

Imagine every step in the daily routine of your "best self." This should be more than the choices your best self makes but also how it feels to be that person. Tying your goals to feelings makes the goals feel more attainable.

Here are some questions to start thinking about who your best self would be:

Morning

How does your best self feel in the morning?

What does your best self do each morning?

What time does she wake up?

What does she eat for breakfast?

Does she work out?

Write down three feelings associated with this morning routine.

Work

What does your best self do for work?

How did she get this job?

How does she interact with her boss?

What does she do at work to make her successful?

Write down three feelings associated with this working life.

Evening

What does she come home to after work?

How does she nourish her body when she gets home?

Does she work out after work?

What time does she go to sleep?

Write down three feelings associated with this evening routine.

If you're a visually creative person, you can also create a vision board. Cut and paste magazine clippings on a poster board or make one on Pinterest using images that evoke your dream life.

What I notice about myself when I do the "Who Is Your Best Self?" exercise is the lack of negative emotions I often feel when trying to reach my goals. Rather than waking up dreading my morning workout, my best self finds a workout that she is excited to get to. Rather than feeling riddled with anxiety before giving a big presentation, when I'm my best self, I feel a sense of assuredness and confidence. It is essential to target these emotions and feelings because they will keep you anchored as you begin a journey to your best self.

Once you have determined, or started to understand, who your best self is, let's combine it with one final step of Hot Girl Walk *As If*. Visualizing is a lot of fun, but you need to take that energy with you throughout your whole day and continue making good and confident decisions.

Many people try to reach goals by punishing themselves for mistakes they've made, which has an inverse effect. For example, I used to put myself on a restrictive diet whenever I wanted to lose weight. When I inevitably broke my diet (it never lasted more than a day), I would overcompensate by skipping a meal or working out extra hard the next day. But this overcompensation would lead me to eat unhealthily, thus beginning a negative cycle. Here, the punishment took me further away from my goals and had a negative impact on my mental health.

However, when I instead imagined myself as my best self, I treated my body differently and no longer limited myself to overly restrictive diets. My best self would never feel guilty for enjoying a meal. She would stick to her regular exercise routine without feeling the need to overcompensate. In this scenario, I make healthy choices out of respect for my body, not out of punishment.

This mindset reduced a lot of the pressure I often placed on myself as a type A individual. With less pressure to succeed, I can focus on the journey, which sets me up for making long-lasting change.

Ask Yourself

Here are some more questions to ask when figuring out who your best self is.

Does the person you want to be:

Stay up late at night stressing before going into an interview?

> No, she feels prepared in her materials and qualifications. She gets a good night's sleep—knowing how important sleep is—to be on her A game.

Skip her workout?

> No, she loves working out. Even though she doesn't want to work out right now, she knows her favorite TV show will be there when she's done, and she'll feel amazing that she stuck to her goal.

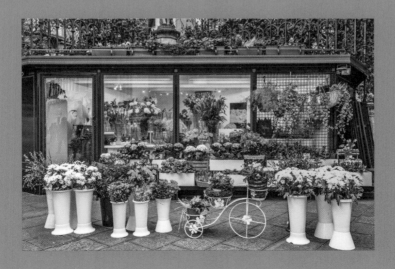

SMART Goals

Once you have a vision of what your future could be, you need to create an actionable plan to achieve that life. The best way to do that is to set one goal, *just one*, and start working toward it now. You may have learned, in school or at work, about the methodology of SMART goals. But if this is the first time you have heard of it, here is the breakdown:

SMART goals are goals that are:

Specific: A specific goal keeps your sights set on something concrete. Just saying, "I want to be successful," is more of a wish than a goal. Dig deeper into what you want to be successful in. Can you narrow down an area of your life where you are seeking this success? Instead of making such a broad statement, your goal should be separate and distinct from the bigger picture.

Measurable: Placing a quantity to a goal makes it measurable. Being able to measure your progress toward your goal is the best way to ensure that you will be able to achieve it. If you ever see your progress plummeting, you have the opportunity to make adjustments and get yourself back on the right path.

Achievable: As much as I love dreaming big, you need achievable goals. In many cases, this means breaking down the steps you need to take. Setting a goal that is too far out of reach can be demotivating and make you feel like you never can meet your goals. Once you can find that starting point, that first step, the path toward achieving your goals becomes that much more tangible.

Relevant: To make your goal relevant means to make sure that it aligns with your long-term vision. When your goal brings you closer to the future you desire, you'll find you're more willing to make it happen. In other words, don't make goals that don't inspire or excite you.

Timely: Lastly, placing a time constraint on your goal can help you take action. Setting a due date, deadline, or end date—whatever you want to call it—will give you a finish line that you can see in the distance. It may be far away, but it is reachable. I know I previously said that the pressure of success often gets in our way. So, when you set this deadline, choose one that is comfortable but optimistic. It shouldn't be too far away, but it also shouldn't be so close that it causes you stress.

SMART Goals Template

Set three SMART goals right now using this template:

Starting [start date] I will [goal] by [end date].

Make these SMART goals your starting point. Check in each week, each month, and each year. Be sure to also track your progress with short-term benchmarks. This can help you stay motivated and on task to reach your goal. Celebrating the small steps taken is essential in keeping you focused on your long-term goal.

Making and Breaking **Habits**

SMART goals are a great way to make actionable steps towards larger goals. If you've tried SMART goals before and want to go about goal achievement in a different way, or if you'd like to add more goals using a different method, another tool I like to utilize deals with making and replacing habits. Where SMART goals can help you focus on large life goals, making new habits can help you achieve smaller lifestyle changes, making you 1 percent better each day.

Many understand habits in the context of bad habits, like biting your nails, for example. But there are also good habits you can start doing that will help improve your life. Before we get started on replacing bad habits, let's first break down what habits are.

Habits are made of three stimuli: trigger, action, and response. Let's use the example of biting your nails. The trigger could be (in most cases) stress; the action is biting your nails; then the reward is that momentary feeling of comfort or control, as is the case in most stressful situations where there is a sense of loss of control.

I've found that a huge barrier holding adults back from living as their best selves is a bad habit associated with stress. Being able to identify a bad habit and replace it or build a new habit to combat it is the first step to creating a lifestyle that fits your best self.

I am not a nail-biter, but I am a chronic snacker. When I was working from home in my corporate job, I developed a snacking habit. When I got stressed at work (trigger), I would get up from my computer and walk 10 feet (3 m)

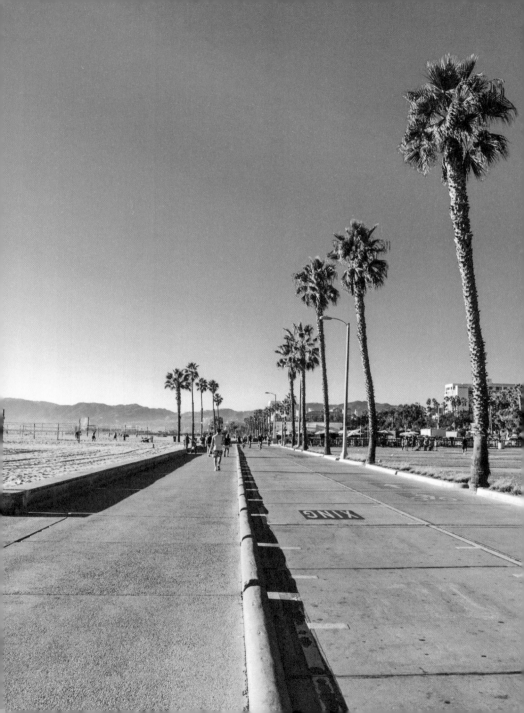

to my kitchen to make a snack (action) as a distraction. This snack was never healthy. I was searching for an instant hit of dopamine to make me feel better during a stressful situation. And my go-to snacks to get that hit were potato chips or chocolates.

After a few months of this cycle, I developed a habit. My brain no longer needed to consider what to do when I became stressed at work. In other words, my brain developed an automatic response to this trigger: Whenever I was stressed at work, I'd immediately feel the need to grab a snack, no matter if I was hungry or not. Shortly thereafter, I would associate working with snacking. Unfortunately, I'm not a professional eater, so this was not what I would consider a productive habit, and I knew something had to change.

My solution was to replace chronic snacking with—you guessed it—Hot Girl Walks. By shifting my mindset to associate work stress with going on a Hot Girl Walk, I was able to give my brain a productive break from work. On my walks, I found the opportunity to gather perspective on whatever was making me stressed, so that when I got back to my desk, I had a clear head to face it and finish my workday.

Making and replacing habits is in no way easy to do, but there are four methods I used that I hope will also help you replace your bad habits:

1 **Habit stacking.** Habit stacking is where you place your desired habit on top of your current habit instead of trying to quit cold turkey. In my case, I was replacing my chronic snacking with Hot Girl Walks. This meant that when I reached for my obligatory 3 p.m. stress-snack, instead of sitting down and eating it, I would take it with me on a short ten-to-twenty-minute Hot Girl Walk. This way I was still enjoying my snack, while also forming a connection between work stress and walking. Eventually, I found myself wanting to go on my walk immediately, and the habit of grabbing a snack slowly slipped away.

2 **Temptation bundling.** Temptation bundling is wrapping up your desired habit with an action you *want*. I used this for my after-work bad habit, which was plopping on my couch and watching my favorite TV show or scrolling on TikTok. Since walking was a new habit I wanted to do more often, I brought this activity onto the treadmill. To make this bundle a bit more manageable, I designated specific shows to watch while walking. So, if I wanted to know what happened next, I needed to take a Hot Girl Walk! Other times, I would bribe myself with getting a fancy latte at a nearby coffee shop on my walk. This is what is called an extrinsic motivator: something that helps you get on your feet when you're first creating a new habit, and your motivation is slowly becoming intrinsic. The Hot Girl Walks you used to take only to go get an expensive croissant will soon become your favorite part of your day even without the sweet treat!

3 **Make it easy.** Make your desired habit the easy choice. Remove all barriers between you and your desired habit. I work from home, so I love to spend my workday in my Hot Girl Walk athleisure. I leave my sneakers by the front door and have a Hot Girl Walk "go bag" (a belt bag that is perpetually filled with anything and everything I could ever need while on the road). All these little things eliminate the amount of effort I need to go through to get out on my Hot Girl Walk. Even the smallest distraction of picking out an outfit or looking for a favorite lip balm could make or break a new habit.

4 **Identify.** Make your new habit a part of your identity. I never saw myself as an athlete, so when I was working out, I always felt intimidated or like an imposter at the gym. Knowing this, when I started the Hot Girl Walk, I found a large community of people who used walking as their main form of exercise. Now, we host community Hot Girl Walks where hundreds of Hot Girl Walk-ers meet and go on a walk together. I confidently consider myself an athlete now.

The key to goal setting is knowing that the finish line shouldn't be the most important thing. Oftentimes, when I start working on a goal, I don't hit it exactly as I had planned to. At the risk of sounding cliché, it *is* more about the journey than the destination. Fall in love with the process of achieving your goals. If you dread every single day of trying, change your strategy. The Hot Girl Walk method is about empowering you to find what works best *for you*.

My final piece of advice answers my most-asked question: What do you do on days when you're not motivated?

In short: I remember that motivation does not exist.

Actually, motivation does exist, but it is fleeting. I used to rely on motivation to carry me as I aimed for ambitious goals. The first few days were always the best. I was excited to achieve whatever I set out to do. But I would never see progress immediately, and after the first few days, my motivation would taper off. As one rest day turned into two, then turned into a week, I'd inevitably throw in the towel and give up.

Discipline is what shows up when motivation is the unreliable friend. Discipline is determining the difference between needing rest and making an excuse. Growing up taking dance classes, I was often pushed further than I should have been pushed, but it was because until you go too far, you don't know your limits. Set expectations for yourself and deliver on those expectations. Much of having confidence is having trust in yourself that you will show up when you say that you will. There is no bigger confidence builder than achieving a goal that you worked to achieve. Discipline is all about realizing that the only person you are doing this for is you. So why choose to let yourself down?

Using these tools to form achievable goals, my best self is no longer an idea or a vision board. Instead, I can see my best self *becoming* myself.

Do the Impossible

I like to do one "impossible" physical task a week. This could be taking a hard hike, trying a daunting fitness class, doing the StairMaster, or going on an extra-long Hot Girl Walk. When I push myself physically, I encounter those thoughts that tell me to "give up." But with the simple knowledge that I am trying to do something I once deemed "impossible," I am prepared to meet that voice, push through, and complete whatever task I've given myself. There is only one person who will get me up the mountain; there is no room to credit anyone else for this achievement. Working out is your opportunity to fail and your opportunity to achieve at no consequence. It's an opportunity to try something new, and if you hate it, don't go back, but at least you can say you tried.

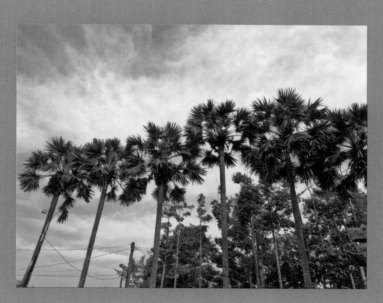

Inspired by
Desiree's Story

When it comes to creating a new habit, it can be challenging to start something so different from our identities. It's part of the reason I always struggled in the fitness world. I would define myself as a "dancer." I was not an "athlete," nor was I a "runner." So, when I tried to do activities that required running or anything else athletic, it always made me feel like a poser. In the gym, I'd feel people staring at me as I huffed and puffed through my twelve-minute mile (it was almost as if I could hear their inner monologue: *She doesn't belong here . . . she's not a runner.*).

Years later, well into my Hot Girl Walk journey, I resumed running, and I even ran a half-marathon. There was a local running club nearby that seemed like the perfect opportunity to meet new people after I graduated college. Maybe they'd lend me some running tips so I wouldn't be lost on the day of my half-marathon (I had never been to a race before, so I needed some advice). But then I scrolled through their Instagram page and felt intimidated. I was now running seven-minute miles with ease, but I could still hear the voice in my head: *She doesn't belong here . . . she's not a runner.*

Desiree had a similar feeling of nervousness before her first Hot Girl Walk:

66 During the first HGW I attended in Santa Monica I was very nervous and self-conscious. But I saw so many women there who looked like me that it made me feel better. Hot Girl Walks have allowed me to create bonds with other women and expand my circle of friends by creating an uplifting community. I'm so proud of myself for putting myself out there and attending a Hot Girl Walk.

My best piece of advice for other people starting their Hot Girl Walk journeys is to be proud of what you can achieve. Even just thirty minutes of walking can make a difference in a month."

I started hosting Hot Girl Walks to make it clear to people who'd find us on Instagram that there are no requirements to join—they are always free and for all skill levels; Hot Girl Walks really are for *everybody*.

Desiree now regularly attends Hot Girl Walks in Los Angeles. This story exemplifies the importance of having a community that is inclusive and accessible to all. When you join the Hot Girl Walk community, you become a Hot Girl Walk-er. Though we meet monthly, that identity sticks with you every day. It is the difference between taking one Hot Girl Walk a month and Hot Girl Walk-ing every day.

EMBRACING SELF-APPRECIATION

Recognizing
Your **Worth**

I started dancing at thirteen years old. If you know anything about dance, most people start as soon as they can walk. After years as a cheerleader, I wanted to change my path and join the dance team as I entered high school. I envied their sparkly outfits and wanted to trade my pom-poms in for a pair of pointe shoes. I mean, what young girl doesn't want to be a ballerina?

When it came time to train for my audition for my high school's dance team, I had to start as a beginner. Ballet is the foundation of most Western dance, so I chose to start there, shoving myself into a tiny leotard that showed a lot more than the T-shirt and Soffe shorts I was used to wearing at cheer practice.

Ballet is an endless pursuit of perfection. Of course, starting at square one, I had a long way to go. Learning the French words, pushing my feet into pointed toes, and asking my sister to sit on my knees before bed so I could have the overextension all ballerinas vie for.

In my area, there were no classes for teenage beginners, so I joined classes for eight- to ten-year-olds. As you can probably imagine, as an already self-conscious teenager, this amplified my self-criticism. Every day after school, with my end goal in mind, I would force myself to show up and train with these young kids, who were much better than I was. It was, for lack of a better term, awkward. I felt so out of place, and even the kids in my classes would tell me if they thought I was bad or if I was doing something wrong.

Luckily, I moved up and out of these classes and was able to make the junior varsity high school dance team. However, I'm a perfectionist. I was so aware

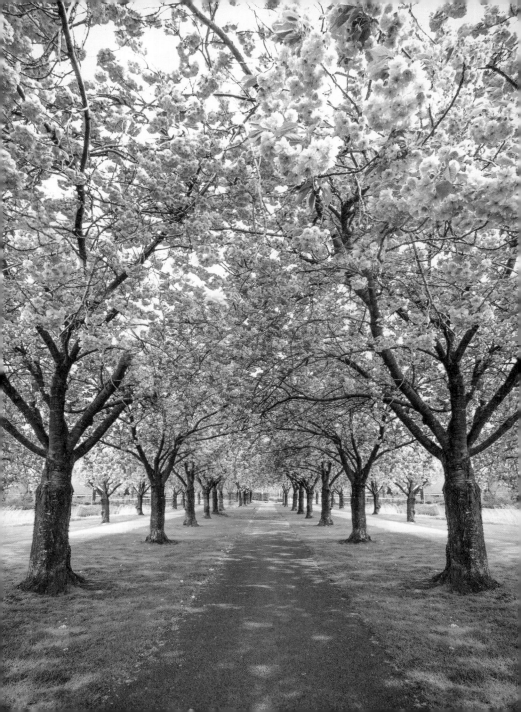

of everything I could be better at. It was this awareness that allowed me to improve faster than my peers, but it also held me back in ways I didn't expect. When it came to the technique, I was focused, dedicated, and determined to be perfect . . . but when it came to the actual movement, I was stunted by my confidence.

All throughout high school, I was often criticized for my lack of confidence because I held my emotions on my face, and it was clear to everybody watching that I did not believe myself to be a dancer. I spent years fixating on my technique and watching other dancers, trying to emulate them. But when it came time to perform, I looked awkward. There were other girls on my dance team who had worse technique than I did but were more fun to watch dance because they had *confidence*. In tight, uncomfortable clothes, I always felt, no matter how hard I worked, that I was not good enough.

It was a little bit of a chicken-and-egg debacle. I felt that if I were a good enough dancer, confidence would come to me. I don't know the exact day when it happened, but I eventually became good enough. Yet I was still waiting for my confidence to set in. It was here that I realized that I couldn't let confidence *happen* to me. I had to grab it and wear it myself, even if it felt like it didn't fit quite right. Back when I was learning with a younger age group, I had the passion and determination to make the dance team, and it was this passion that drove me to push past any embarrassment. While this confidence felt uncomfortable most of the time, it helped me reach my goal.

Defying the Odds

Join me in remembering a moment that you took a leap, no matter the cost. It can be small or large. Pick the first moment that sticks out in your mind; reach out and grab it, so we can take a closer look. It's OK if it takes some time to come to you. Take your time. There's no rush. I also encourage you to utilize this exercise as a journal prompt. Writing these feelings and thoughts down helps make them metaphorically concrete.

Once you have that moment, answer the following questions:

> **How old were you? Maybe you were young or maybe it was just last year. An estimate will work here.**
>
> **What was the scenario? What were you trying to achieve?**
>
> **Why were you so determined to get there? Was it something you'd had your eye on for a long time, or was it something that you knew you had to do at that period of your life?**
>
> **What obstacles did you have to cross? Of these obstacles, which were the most challenging?**
>
> **Did you have any doubts in your mind when encountering these obstacles?**
>
> **What did you do to push through these doubts and overcome them?**
>
> **What feelings did you have when you achieved your task? Or if you didn't, how did you feel?**
>
> **Did you learn something new about yourself? What was it that you learned?**
>
> **Are you glad you went on that journey?**

Recognize the strength that comes with pushing past the odds to go for something you're passionate about. Recognize how positively you think and/ or write about this past version of yourself—the person who faced hardship but persevered regardless of success. This person is very much a part of you, and you deserve the same grace and reverence. Moments of perseverance are always so much clearer in the future, so give yourself that space. Now, take that confidence and wear it every day.

My lack of confidence affected not only my dance but other areas of my life, such as public speaking, dating, and applying to colleges and jobs. I was so insecure about myself that I didn't trust myself and it showed in my style, my performance in interviews, and so much more. Not trusting myself forced me to make choices based on what I *thought* I should do, which only felt more uncomfortable. Becoming confident became my only focus.

Rather than studying how people dressed, ate, or what they did, I instead started studying their intrinsic "why," such as how they thought and how they spoke about themselves. I started mimicking their confidence. They say practice makes perfect, and I found that to be true for confidence as well. I took "fake it till you make it" to another level and let the extrinsic confidence seep into my intrinsic beliefs.

The challenge was to practice my confidence in intervals. If I had a big interview, I would speak like I was the most confident girl in the world, as if I had a lot of achievements to be proud of. It felt uncomfortable, but I told myself, *It's just thirty minutes. You can freak out for the rest of the day but just put it on for thirty minutes.*

The more I talked about my achievements as they deserved to be talked about, I started to feel my confidence lasting past thirty minutes. Instead of saying, "I just did some leadership at my sorority, but it was during COVID," it became, "I was president of my sorority while navigating a challenging time." I realized I had a negative view of my accomplishment and therefore a negative view of myself. My accomplishments were never enough for me, so when I tried to communicate them in an interview, they never came across as a benefit of my character.

Activities for the Treadmill

The moment I realized I had reached a new echelon of confidence was when I felt comfortable doing things on my own, such as going to the gym, going out to dinner, or even just exploring my city. I never knew how a lack of confidence inhibited my life until I realized how rare it was that I spent time doing things by myself. As much as I loved spending time with friends and family, I found I was overly reliant on the people around me, and I didn't know what it was like to just be by myself.

Now, I enjoy doing things alone, even being so brazen as to watch my favorite shows on the treadmill at the gym. In fact, the people at the gym now know me as "the girl with the iPad." This fact would have humiliated me in the past, but slowly, more people began telling me that they bought iPads so they could watch TV on the treadmill too.

Instead of waiting for my friends to be available, I take myself to new areas and restaurants in my city. On these mini solo adventures, I've made so many memories and even met new friends.

Small moments like these have made the biggest difference in my life and my newfound confidence. I've seen bigger lifestyle changes like a healthier diet, joy in exercising, and being more sociable. These thirty-minute stints of confidence, these mini moments all compiled together, have taken the biggest weight off my shoulders.

Here are more situations where I've used thirty minutes of confidence to get me through:

* Scheduling a doctor's appointment
* Telling my server that my order is wrong
* Having fun at karaoke night
* Meeting new people without minimizing my personality
* Proudly communicating my accomplishments in an interview

If you find yourself encountering these situations with a lack of confidence, know that you are not alone, but that it's also up to you to change your approach. To make progress, you need to believe in yourself. Trust yourself to work through your emotions and be successful in everything you set out to do.

Gaining a
Self-Confident
Glow

As I mentioned in an earlier chapter, confidence is having trust in yourself that you will accomplish what you set out to do. Having trust in yourself is what differentiates you from everybody else. When you admire a celebrity for their style or unique look, it's often because they dare to be different from everybody else. They have trust in their style instincts and make choices that suit them rather than suit expectations.

Self-confidence brings what I call a "glow." It's a power that comes from inside you and emanates outward. It's little choices like avoiding the latest fad to try your own thing or choosing to not follow a makeup trend because you know what makes *you* beautiful. Take a leap and don't be afraid to be different.

Find Your Glow

Many times, we let our success wash past us. This exercise is meant to help you identify your best qualities that you may not fully trust or give yourself enough credit for. Identify these traits and let them make you shine brighter!

Answer the following questions. It's time to set aside your modesty and be honest about how great you are. Find somewhere to write down these answers so that you never forget and for when you need a reminder.

* When was the last time you felt strong?
* What were you doing at that moment?
* When was the last time you felt confident? What were you doing, wearing, thinking about? What was the precise moment that made you realize this confidence?
* When was the last time you felt proud? What did you do that made you feel proud?
* When was the last time you felt truly special? What about this moment sticks out in your mind?
* What can you do to replicate these feelings of strength, confidence, pride, and uniqueness in your daily life?

This exercise is meant to give you strength and build trust behind the traits that make you most special. With a more solid connection between you and these traits, you should feel more confident to dive into what makes *you uniquely you.*

Methods to *Acknowledge* Your Worth

Confidence stems from how you view yourself, starting with how you internally speak about yourself. The Mean Mia I mentioned earlier was my biggest critic. She would call me "stupid," "ugly," and "out of shape" without needing any evidence to make me believe it. Nobody else in my life spoke to me like this, and if someone tried, I would fight back. So why was it so different in my own head?

Studies show that if you put a pencil horizontally between your teeth, mimicking a smile, you're more likely to be happy. There are tricks we can do with our bodies to persuade our minds into believing something is true. Standing up a little taller when you feel insecure may feel dissonant to your mind, but soon enough your brain will catch on.

Start by changing your external monologue, and eventually your internal monologue will follow. It sounds easier than it is, I know. When I first started doing this, I viewed it as a joke. I would get an *A* on my paper, and I would say to my friends, "Obviously, I'm a genius!" I'd get asked out on a date and

I'd say, "Obviously, I'm beautiful!" My friends and I all spoke like this, agreeing with each other that we had so much to be proud of . . . though our words had an undercurrent of hyperbole and satire.

But it felt good. Speaking about myself in a positive way and then having my friends hype me up worked. I slowly adopted the word "obviously" as my new mantra. I heard Mean Mia getting quieter and quieter as this new Confident Mia emerged in my head. And I started to believe in myself.

You can create a mantra of your own to help turn your internal monologue from mean to uplifting. Make it a routine and say it to yourself in the mirror before work or school. Create a muscle in your brain that says this mantra when times are tough. Start with just two words: I am . . . I am smart, talented, confident, and kind. Write it on your hand or make yourself a friendship bracelet with those words on it. Say it every day, say it when life is challenging, say it when you don't believe it.

Hot Thoughts

Write down ten traits that you like about yourself on sticky notes and place them on your mirror. I call these traits "powers." Every day, look yourself in the eye, and remind yourself of your powers that make you a Hot Girl.

Each week, pick one power to celebrate and practice. So often, in our jobs, we aren't able to flex our favorite powers. For example, if your power is "I am creative," go do something to flex that creative muscle, perhaps by sitting in the park and drawing. If your power is "I am beautiful," take yourself to get a facial or break out the workout set you've been saving for an extra special Hot Girl Walk.

I talked about the power of gratitude in the first chapter, but I want to make it very clear that you should not be grateful for your achievements. Instead, I want you to take ownership of them. When we dilute our success by giving false credit to others, we take away our own power.

When I got into USC through my appeal letter, it should have felt like a huge accomplishment, but I still have a hard time talking about it because I didn't feel like I really earned it. Instead, I accredited luck to my acceptance. I worked every day to feel like I was worthy of being at college and overachieved while I was there. I stacked up my achievements, but it still wasn't enough. After spending my whole life expecting my power to fall in my lap, I had to learn how to grab it. Once I started *taking* credit for my achievements, I believed in my power and finally began to wear my confidence.

You must be your biggest cheerleader. Only you know how great you are, and how much greater you *will* be.

When I think back to that first dance class, I used to imagine everyone was staring at me and just waiting for me to fail. Until I finally realized: they were all too busy looking at their own reflections in the mirror. Stop looking at everyone else. Instead of making a vision board with pictures of celebrities, turn it into a mirror. Don't spend your time envying what other people have that you don't. Focus on the power you already have inside.

HIIT Confidence Practice

Challenge yourself to be the most confident version of yourself for ten minutes. Even if you feel like it doesn't fit, it's just ten minutes. Leave all your doubt for outside those ten minutes and allow your confidence to linger as long as it can.

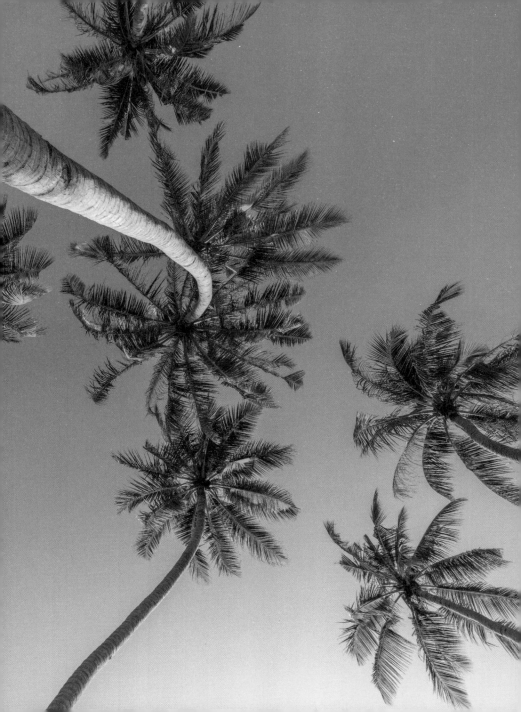

Inspired by
Heather's Story

Confidence was something that I had to develop on my own. I always expected it to come from someone else and would seek external validation. Yet time and time again, it would never fix my insecurities. Using the tools above, I trained myself to be confident. It was like a muscle that had atrophied, and I had to retrain it to grow stronger. Starting Hot Girl Walk taught me a lot about confidence, but I've also learned a lot from the people I've met in this community.

Heather comes to the Hot Girl Walks in New York City. Heather is the kind of person people gravitate toward, someone who is beautiful from the inside out. Here's what Hot Girl Walk means to her:

> **I recently lost 60 pounds, and Hot Girl Walk has been my way of connecting with nature. It's a chance to be outside and be surrounded by amazing women. My favorite Hot Girl Walk memories are watching the autumn leaves fall and singing 'Man, I Feel Like a Woman' walking around Central Park.**
>
> **I have told all my friends about Hot Girl Walk events and it's been a great way to connect and see each other at least once a month.**

My best piece of advice is that the hardest part is starting, but then moving your body becomes the food for your soul."

Hot Girl Walk-ing around Central Park, blasting Shania Twain, hanging with your girlfriends: that is the picture of confidence. When we are able to take care of ourselves and can "feed our souls," this becomes an energy inside of you that has no choice but to glow for the world to see. Finding moments like this in our lives is the key to confidence. With a village surrounding us, there is a sense of invincibility, a feeling that we can't be touched or hurt. This village gives us the confidence to be our truest selves.

BUILDING

RESIL

IENCE

Overcoming *Challenges*

I am more confident than I ever have been in my life, and confidence never came naturally to me. It was something I had to work toward and practice. With that being said, I am not confident *all* the time. In fact, quitting my corporate job to start a business at twenty-four years old was the biggest test of the skills I have developed with Hot Girl Walk.

Not only was I starting my business young, but I launched it on social media, which meant that everyone had something to say. Whether it was their thoughts on Hot Girl Walk to how I look or speak, it's all open to public opinion. Beyond social media, I have received unwarranted criticism from people in the industry.

Had I started posting on social media even a few months sooner than I did, it would have irrevocably damaged the views I had of myself. Hot Girl Walks are my therapy. They keep me sane no matter what comes my way. However, this isn't the case all the time; when I first started, the fear of my negative thought cycle held me back from walking in the first place.

It was on my Hot Girl Walks that I really homed in on a strategy for defeating my negative thoughts. Strategy is important because your negative thoughts will never disappear completely—they are there for a reason. Building a strategy to overcome negativity will make you stronger and more resilient in the future.

On a Hot Girl Walk, your mind has to be a judgement free zone. There are many elements of mindfulness that you can practice on your Hot Girl Walk. The goal here is to make the biggest element not berating yourself for having these thoughts. This way you can adjust the emotions you feel as a result.

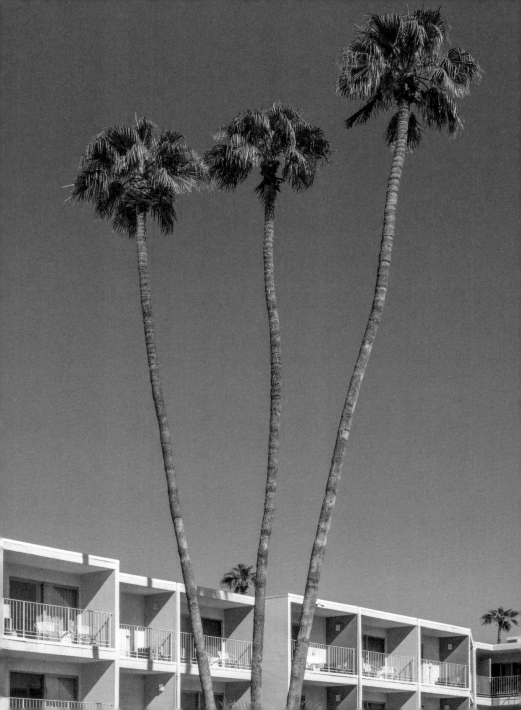

The Tornado *of* Negativity

A negative spiral is when your emotions are disproportionate to the circumstance itself. Imagine this negative spiral as a tornado. The top, or wide opening, of the storm is what is actually happening to you. As you start to deliberate and anticipate what will happen next, you move closer to the eye of the storm, and as the wind picks up, so do the negative thoughts, such as your poor reactions and inability to accomplish whatever this circumstance represents. The situation then becomes clouded by self-judgment until it is all that you can see. In other words, your negative thoughts dictate these experiences, and you create low self-confidence in yourself.

Here's an example of what this can look like:

"I can't believe I flunked that physics exam."

"Well, maybe if I had studied harder, I wouldn't have failed."

"I don't deserve to be at my university if I can't study hard enough to pass my exam."

"I should drop out of university because I didn't pass."

"I am a failure."

We know that failing one exam doesn't make you a failure or require dropping out of college. Reading this now with a clear head, that is obvious. But it's hard to think clearly when you're stuck in a tornado of negativity because your feelings are so strong. Recognizing that you're spiraling can be the first step to coming out of it.

While it's important to be able to recognize your negative spiral, it's even more important not to judge it. You can easily slip into the thought pattern of, *Not only am I a failure, but I'm negative too!* Everybody gets themselves into these thinking paradoxes, and it's a major reason why many people, including myself, can be afraid of being alone with their thoughts.

After recognizing and not judging a negative spiral, I jump back into my gratitude practice (see Cultivating Gratitude, page 22). This allows my emotions to level out while my mind is distracted by doing something concrete.

Recognizing a Negative Spiral

Think of a time when you've encountered a circumstance that made you feel really bad about yourself. A failed test, a mistake at work, messing up on a speech: these small mistakes can be blown out of proportion in your mind.

Ask yourself: What were your initial thoughts? What did you do in reaction to those thoughts? What could you have done instead to combat the negative thoughts and encourage yourself to do better next time?

If this situation happens again, how will you resist going through another tornado of negativity? Come up with actionable steps that you know help boost your spirits and break the cycle.

Personifying
Your *Negative*
Thoughts

Here's a simple exercise to recognize your negative spiral: personify your negative thoughts, as if they're friends talking to you. I've found that turning intense emotions into an entity that is receptive to your thoughts and words makes it easier to talk them out and argue against them. I know I would tell a good friend these thoughts are irrational, but sometimes when we are up against ourselves, those are the hardest voices to combat.

You may remember our friend Mean Mia, which is my nickname for my negative inner voice. I have personified my negative thoughts as someone else saying them to me. This way, I can separate myself in two and have a conversation with Mean Mia to try to understand what she may be trying to say underneath all those harsh words.

Personifying my negative thoughts has helped me realize there were no grounds for these beliefs I had about myself. I realized all these negative beliefs were based on a desire to be the best version of myself. If I ever thought, *I am so dumb because I messed up this task at work*, that thought was inspired by my feeling that *I know I can do better*. But instead of sugarcoating these thoughts, my internal monologue knew the quickest way to knock me down.

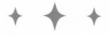

The other things I used to hear Mean Mia saying were based on my anxieties: *That mistake you made is going to get you fired*. This is an extreme thought that blows the circumstance out of proportion. Mean Mia is looking out for me. She wants me to be my best self and doesn't want me caught off guard if the worst scenario happens. While we need to honor these thoughts, we cannot let ourselves fall victim to them.

Goodbye, Negativity!

Once you identify these thoughts and what your negative internal monologue is trying to say to you, start responding with this simple acknowledgment: *Thank you for letting me know. I know you have my best interest at heart but dwelling on the negative won't bring a positive.*

Say this aloud or in your head as many times as you need to and walk away from your own Mean Mia. When you go on a Hot Girl Walk, imagine that each step is walking away from these negative thoughts.

Law of
Attraction

Negative thoughts breed negative action. If you focus on negativity, you will end up making a negative thought real. This is the "Law of Attraction." The Law of Attraction is the principle of positive thoughts breeding positive results and vice versa for negative thoughts. Some people find this to be a spiritual belief and even call it "manifestation." I am very much rooted in action over manifestation, but the Law of Attraction has some evidence in psychology.

We went over the self-fulfilling prophecy phenomenon in an earlier chapter, and the Law of Attraction has a similar moral. A self-fulfilling prophecy is where you let your beliefs influence your actions, which results in a fear coming true. The Law of Attraction has a broader cause and effect: The negative beliefs that you have will bring negativity towards you. However, if you put out positive thoughts and actions, positive things will come to you.

Whether or not you believe in a karmic equilibrium in the universe, it's largely understood that our minds persevere over matter. The Law of Attraction does not explain why bad things happen to good people. Sometimes negativity occurs that is beyond our control. This is why we must have resilience to persevere when life throws us challenges.

Pull Back and Look In

One of my professors in college gave me this exercise. It was meant for a corporate environment, but I have found that it's worked in many other areas of my life. She said, "When something bad has happened at work—maybe someone spoke out of line or made a crucial error that your boss blamed you for—you need to pull back and look in." You may feel the desire to write a scathing email or storm into your boss's office, but instead you need to take these two steps:

Pull Back: Imagine yourself soaring outside of your body and take a third-person perspective of the scenario. In other words, remove yourself from your emotions and look at the situation objectively or professionally.

Look In: Now that you have an unbiased view of your situation, you should be able to understand what happened, what is going on, and what the next steps are.

When things happen outside of our control, they may be jarring and spur us to act immediately. This exercise forces us to look outside of our circumstances.

Imagine what it looks like when it's raining. When you're underneath the rain cloud, it looks like—no matter where you are—the entire world is being rained on, and everything is covered in a gray sheet. But when you are outside the rain cloud, you can see that the rain is not so universal, and the cloud will pass.

Hot Girl Walks are *essential* to the "pull back, look in" approach. When you are at work, school, or surrounded by negative thoughts, they can seem all-consuming. Taking a step back forces you into a new perspective. You realize that the world is still turning, though when you are inside, it seems like the world is ending. Maybe you start to see people going about their days with their own challenges and struggles to deal with too. Let this new perspective soothe you and keep you from falling into that negative spiral.

Now that you have pulled back and looked deeper into your circumstances, you may, at the very least, have let your emotions calm down. Responding with heightened emotions can be detrimental, so I try to avoid this at all costs. If I can sleep on an email, I do. Many times, we aren't given that luxury, though, and we have to respond quickly. In such cases, I immediately pull back and look in, and maybe even send my email to a trusted friend to read over before responding. You have the control to stop yourself from posting or sending anything you could regret.

When I was president of my sorority, situations like this would happen often. I would immediately get hot and want to defend myself and fight back. I knew, however, that fighting back would only fan the flames. Though I may have been shaking with rage, I would take a deep breath and address it when my mind was clearer.

This approach can also provide clarity when personal obstacles arise. Unfortunately, you cannot Hot Girl Walk your way out of many challenges life throws at you. But it does feel great to look back at a situation and realize you handled it better than you might've months ago.

Use the previous strategies to keep your mindset strong and remember that gratitude can keep you grounded in the good. What I am still dealing with is the lack of control I feel over obstacles. It's something I know triggers negative emotions, but now I also know how to tackle them whenever they come.

When It Rains, It Doesn't Have to Pour

If you're on a Hot Girl Walk and it starts raining, you have two options: Hot Girl Walk through the rain or call a rideshare and go home. While you can't control the weather, the one thing you can control is how you perceive this obstacle. It can be frustrating that your plan has been derailed, but the frustration you hold in such circumstances can be a heavier weight than the inconvenience was in the first place. You *can* control your response. So don't let the rain stop you from having a good day.

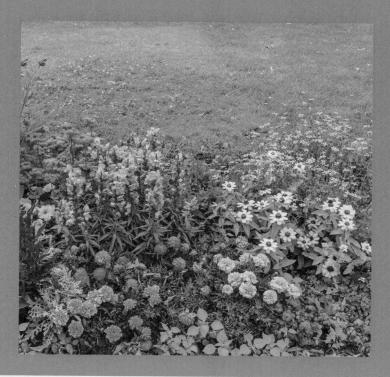

Inspired by
Hilary's Story

Hilary has taught me a vital lesson, though we've never had the chance to meet. She sent me this email, and it put into perspective what it means to control what you can and persevere through obstacles. She wrote:

" I've followed your Hot Girl Walk journey for several years on TikTok. In November, I was hospitalized for twelve days in acute liver failure. It was unexpected; I've been healthy my whole life and have no family history of liver disease, so the whole thing was so shocking and scary. I remember watching your Hot Girl Walks while I was in the hospital and convinced myself to get up and do my own Hot Girl Walks around the acute/oncology unit. At my weakest point, I collapsed in the middle of the unit and had to be carried back to my room. I lay in bed that night and cried and promised myself I would never take walking for granted again. If by some miracle I was able to move forward with my life, I would prioritize walking Hot Girl style. After I regained my strength, I started walking around the unit again, the nurses at each station would high-five me and cheer me on. Eventually I was discharged and continued my journey. Hot Girl Walks around my house led to a lap around my neighborhood, to two laps, to 3 miles and today, I'm able to walk 10 miles every day.

Walking no longer feels like a chore; it is a privilege. I honor it as part of my self-care routine. I know without a doubt it has kept me physically and mentally strong enough to fight this battle for both me and my family.

Your advocacy of walking not only changed but perhaps saved my life. Thank you for being an inspiration and a beacon of hope to women like me."

Hilary's story is nothing short of inspirational. It shows that our response to our circumstances defines us. What Hot Girl Walk offers is an opportunity to defy your situation. It is also a sandbox for you to grow your resilience muscles in. Just like confidence, resilience must be practiced. Although Hilary was going through a challenging time, she had the goal of being able to go on Hot Girl Walks. This goal helped Hilary stay strong physically and mentally during a tough time.

Unfortunately, life can and will throw new challenges our way, whether as an obstacle to a goal or a wrench in our lives. We can only be grateful for our circumstances and recognize that we can overcome hard things.

When I am faced with challenges, I often say to myself, "I have been through worse, and I can survive this." We are always stronger than what we give ourselves credit for.

EMBRACING

ACING

SISTER

HOOD

88

THE POWER OF Community

91

MAKE A Commitment

96

SPEND TIME, EARN Trust

100

BREAK DOWN Walls

The Power of *Community*

Growing up with a younger sister, sisterhood always seemed like a clear concept to me. My mom instilled in us from an early age that our sisterhood eclipsed all our other best friends.

"Your sister is your best friend," my mom would say when I would tell her about my new best friend. It was her way of reminding me that while I was meeting new people, my sister should always come first. No matter what happened—the drama at school, the boys I liked, the trouble I got into—my sister was the person who would stay through it all. And not because she had to. I know how lucky I am to have a good relationship with my siblings. My sister would stay close because our mom raised us to lean on each other.

That's of course not to say that my sister and I didn't fight about the silliest things. But then five minutes would pass, and we'd be hunched over in laughter like nothing ever happened. It's true that a relationship between a blood sister and a relationship between a random girl who becomes your best friend is different, but because of how I was raised as a sister, I would grow to form a deeper respect with the women in my life.

Throughout my life, I found sisterhood in other places. First, it was on my high school dance team, then in my sorority, where we were literally classified as sisters, then with my college roommates, and now with my Hot Girl Walk community. It was not until my corporate job that I realized the importance of sisterhood, especially ones that come in different forms. I never realized how lucky I was to find a sisterhood in so many different areas of my life until I worked in a male-dominated industry, and I struggled to find my footing.

I had created Hot Girl Walk while I was in college, and, when first starting my corporate job, I had no idea where my company would take me. But, as I experienced a lack of sisterhood for the first time in my life, I realized I probably was not alone in this feeling. In college, I enjoyed Hot Girl Walks with friends and sometimes other people would join us. After graduating and working at my company for a few months, I wanted to bring that feeling of sisterhood back into my life. So, I went onto Instagram and asked if people would be interested in joining me on my daily walks. And to my huge surprise, over one hundred people showed up, from old friends whom I hadn't seen in years to complete strangers looking for connection as well.

After that happened, I was lucky enough to also find strong female mentors at my company. It was through this mentorship that I felt as if I was finally able to establish my place and grow.

There's something to be said about forming good working relationships with your coworkers. If you're not happy at your job, you're never going to be motivated to push yourself and reach that next level—whether that's a pay raise, a higher position in your department, or a bigger part in the company. Finding female mentors—that small sisterhood—who took me under their wing and explained why things were the way they were helped create a safe place where I could grow and keep growing. I owe my success at that company to those women who were in my corner and held my hand through the tough times of being a woman in a male-dominated field. I also owe all the Hot Girl Walks that helped me get by after working a full day sat behind a desk.

Hot Girl Walk started as a meditative practice I did by myself, and then it turned into an outlet for community. Our community is full of people who love to get outside and move, but even more so, it is a community of women who empower others. But there were a few steps I had to take to reach this point.

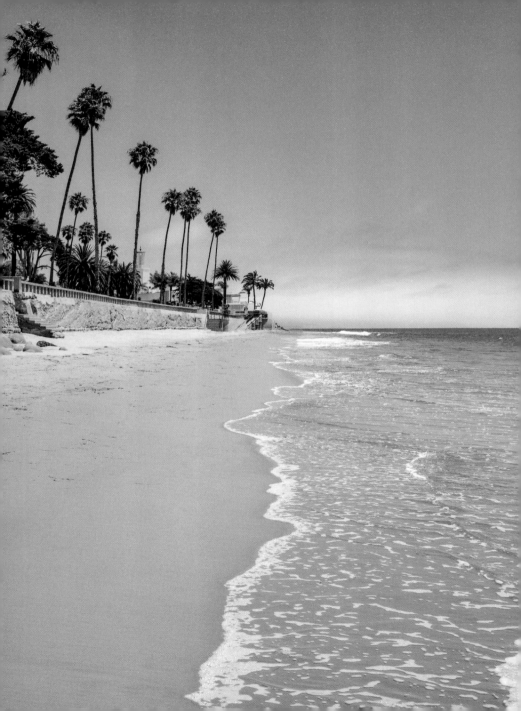

Make *a* Commitment

Commitment is one of the biggest foundations of a successful community. The question I get asked most about hosting Hot Girl Walk events around the world is, "How do you actually make friends?"

Going to events with hundreds of women can be a scary concept, but once you do it enough times and you know exactly what you're walking into and who you're going to meet, that fear turns into more of a nervous anticipation. I've talked to women at my events who've said the big crowd almost made them too scared to get out of their cars. But with a moment of courage, they decided to go for it and ended up enjoying the community they felt while surrounded by all those people. The commitment of showing up is the key to finding and getting the most out of a community. Just like with friends and family, we have to show up, even when we sometimes are not in the mood to do so.

That First Step

Making friends in a new environment—a new school, new job, a running club, a Hot Girl Walk event—can be scary. It can also be scary to be the one to make the first move. It takes a level of vulnerability to essentially say to someone: "You don't know me, I don't know you, but maybe we can be friends!" The good news is, nobody is judging you as hard as you are. We all have feelings of self-consciousness when it comes to meeting new people, and most people are so focused on themselves that they're not worrying about you too.

I used to have a lot of social anxiety: I would get so anxious meeting new people and then replay small blunders I'd make in social interactions. When I finally stopped hyper-fixating on myself, I realized that everyone felt awkward, said things they were embarrassed by, and maybe even stuck their foot in their mouth a few times. All these things that I felt were unique to me were actually things that everyone experienced.

Here's a good affirmation to say to yourself before you make that first step: *I have a lot to offer in a friendship. I'm looking forward to meeting new people, hearing their stories, and making new friends with those who respect me and recognize that I have a lot to offer as a friend.*

This affirmation does two things:

1 It gives you confidence by reminding you that you have a lot of great things about you! You have friends and family who love to spend time with you. It is not your job to mold yourself into someone you think *they* will like. You have something special that only *you* can bring to a relationship.

2 It reminds us that relationships are a two-way street. It removes all the focus we typically place on ourselves, and it makes us present in conversations. It also reminds us we have something to learn from everyone we meet. We recognize the value that we bring to relationships, but does this person also recognize and respect you for this value?

★ **If yes: great!** Most of the time, the people who *want* to meet other people have their hearts open to making new friends. These are the kinds of people I like to have in my life. There is value in every relationship we create, whether it's with a friendly coworker, a friend that you sit next to in class, or just for the day at a Hot Girl Walk.

★ **If not: that's okay.** Not everyone is everyone's cup of tea. There is no use in entering a relationship with someone who doesn't respect you.

At the very least, you put yourself out there, you met someone new, maybe you learned something new about them, and now you can move on. We have all made awkward/bad first impressions, so give this person grace that maybe they are just having a bad day.

The other piece of advice I give to people who ask me how to make friends at a Hot Girl Walk is to just make the first move. Nearly 80 percent of people who attend our events come alone. Even the people who come with friends are there because they want to meet new people. The thing that is so special about this community is that it is grounded in female empowerment, and everyone has such interesting stories to tell. Most of the time, people are just waiting for someone to walk up and introduce themselves, so why can't that be you?

It also helps that everyone is at a Hot Girl Walk event for the same reasons: to walk, to find confidence, and to better their lives. The events are filled with positivity and joy, making it easier to approach strangers because you know everyone is already in a friendly mood. And you already have some things in common to talk about.

While the Hot Girl Walk is grounded in a community of like-minded women, what I find most valuable is the diversity of thought. Social media can force us into echo chambers of ideals and experiences. But in a crowd of people from all walks of life, everyone has a story to share. I like to use our events as an opportunity to find nuggets of wisdom. When you're in a group of hundreds of people, that is an opportunity to open yourself to new perspectives and thoughts. You'd be surprised to find that many people are willing to talk and offer their insights to you. All you need to do is ask.

For instance, at a Hot Girl Walk in Los Angeles, I was leading the pack when a young woman ran up to me and introduced herself. I recognized her name because, as it turned out, we had been going back and forth via direct messages on Instagram for a while now. From our messages, I knew she had been battling cancer, so it was hard for her to show up consistently. However, at this Hot Girl Walk, she let me know she had just "rung the bell" to enter remission from cancer. She spent the entire 4 miles sharing her story with me: how she thought she would never see a light at the end of the tunnel, but even then, she kept fighting to show her two young daughters what strength means. I spent the entire route with tears in my eyes at how empowering her story was.

A few months later, I spent a Hot Girl Walk speaking to a young woman who had moved to California during the pandemic to work with unhoused people. The stories she shared with me about those she met were some of the most powerful stories I have heard to this day.

I never hear the same story twice at a Hot Girl Walk. I collect these stories and learn something new from everyone I speak with; it truly makes me feel grateful to each and every person who followed through on their commitment to show up and made that event so special. Of course, commitment works both ways. If I hadn't started the Hot Girl Walk, if I hadn't continued to host events around the world, then others wouldn't have committed to the movement and found these moments of sisterhood. Like I said at the beginning, sisterhood and community are so important, so whenever you see the opportunity to create them, take it!

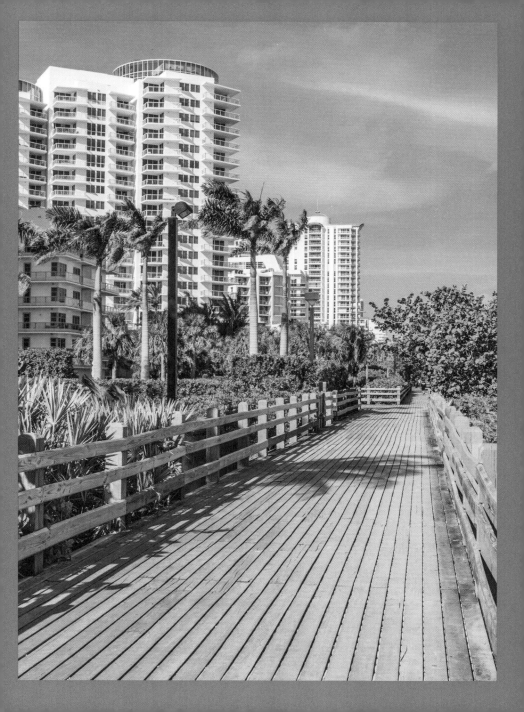

Spend Time, Earn Trust

With all this talk about sisterhood and community, let's not forget that it takes time to build them. It is no easy feat to find people who get along and who will put in constant effort to keep the relationship strong, especially if you're dealing with coworkers where everyone is at a different stage of life. Likewise, if you want to build a community, you need to continuously show up for one another in order to build trust.

Ever since the pandemic, feelings of loneliness have been at an all-time high. I live in Los Angeles, but my Hot Girl Walk events take place around the world. The most common thing I hear at each of these events, which take place in some of the world's biggest cities, is how hard it is to find friends in general. In fact, I can attest to this myself.

I have lived in Los Angeles nearly my entire life. My family moved us from New York when I was seven years old and too young to understand the implications of moving across the country. It wasn't until I started school that it began to sink in. I was "the new kid" and it seemed like everyone had friends already. My mom told me to just go up to people on the playground and say, "Hi, I'm Mia. Do you want to be my friend?" And surprisingly, it worked. So, when I changed schools again in sixth grade, I reused the line and continued to use it all the way through college.

I can't pinpoint the moment when Hot Girl Walks went from monthly get-togethers into a community. One turning moment took place when I was at a grocery store near my apartment and got stopped by someone who recognized me from the Hot Girl Walks. She wanted to let me know that she would come next time. I knew something had changed when we celebrated someone's engagement at another walk, sang happy birthday at another, and began cheering each other on as we hit major milestones.

There is no quick way to create something filled with people you can trust and respect. Trust takes time. Commitment can only be seen as you repeatedly perform the action. All of it takes time. There also isn't one foolproof way to start a new community, like I found with my mom's phrase when I started a corporate job virtually and had trouble making connections with my coworkers. It all depends on the situation and the people, and it will require some trial and error. But if you persist, commit, and show up, that trust will build. And soon you may find yourself surrounded by a community of like-minded people.

As anyone who lives in a bustling city knows, you can be surrounded by a lot of people but still feel alone. That's why we often have *hundreds* of people showing up at our Hot Girl Walk events. The key to building sisterhood is that it isn't just seen—it's felt.

Creating a Community

Community can be found in more places than you may realize. The obvious places are school or work, but your hobbies could become the key to community. One of my friends combined her love of hosting with her roommate's love of reading to start a book club. It started out with a few of their shared friends until we all became a community: celebrating when members got married, became pregnant, or found a new job.

Here are the conditions/steps for creating a community:

★ **Identify an activity.** Maybe it's an existing hobby or one you want to start. An activity is important because shared tasks bond people. They allow our minds to be distracted enough while allowing conversation to flow with ease. The best part is that if you run out of stuff to talk about, you can talk about what you're doing! It should be something accessible as well. If the activity is too difficult or expensive, it's harder to meet consistently. Here are some examples to get you started:

- **A TV show watch party:** Watching TV is something many people do on their own, so it's the perfect vessel for creating community. TV shows air weekly and therefore make their own consistent schedule for a club!

- **Book club:** It's a classic! Each meeting/book can have a different theme, and you can rotate between who chooses the next book. You will learn so much about one another by discussing books.

- **Craft club:** Each meeting can be a new craft. Art is an innately relaxing activity, and each member can agree to rotate hosting. You may surprise yourself, or you may all just have a good laugh at your collective lack of artistic abilities.

Find your people. Invite your friends over and tell them to bring a friend. Maybe use it as an opportunity to invite a person you met once briefly but always wanted to get to know better.

Make a schedule. Showing up week after week, or every other week, becomes ingrained in people's lives. Just like sitting next to Abigail in chemistry class, consistency and repetition can create a bond. Sometimes it takes meeting someone more than once.

Breaking bread. Food is the key to the soul. Sharing snacks or meals has long been the way humans have created bonds and relationships. Try out a new recipe, celebrate birthdays with cupcakes, or share your favorite lasagna recipe that your mom used to make for you. Maybe you'll even learn a few things or find a new favorite food.

⭐ **Lead by example.** In a group of people who may not know each other well, lead by example. Be vulnerable by sharing stories of your own. Facilitate introductions by finding commonalities between people. Listen intently when others speak. Ask a million questions. The openness and closeness of your community starts with you.

Communities like these are the perfect way to break up your week. They make a hump day into Book Club Day and add excitement to your whole week rather than only looking forward to the weekend.

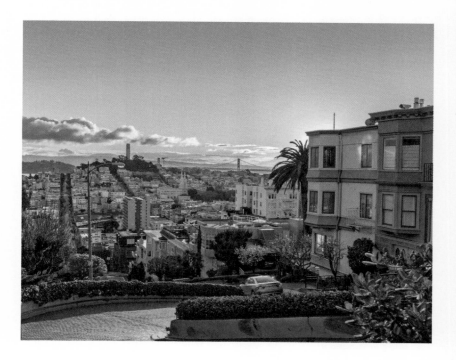

Break *Down* Walls

The first time I hosted a Hot Girl Walk in Miami, my stomach was in knots. It wasn't my first time leading an event or traveling to another city for one either. Perhaps it was because our spots kept filling up, and I had a feeling it would be our biggest event yet. Nonetheless, I knew that I couldn't be nervous because other people would catch my energy. So, I created a cheer the night before over dinner and decided to teach it the next day at the walk.

It took us an hour to check everyone in. We had over five hundred people attend that Hot Girl Walk. It was by far the most people I had ever spoken to. At that point, I had already gotten over my fear of public speaking, but the sea of people staring at me nearly made it return. But once again, I realized that if I was nervous, everyone else would be too. So I decided then and there that it wasn't so serious, and we were all there to have fun. With that confidence, I did what I told myself I was going to do and taught the cheer, hoping people would respond.

I shouted, "Repeat after me! Ain't no walk," and I pointed at the crowd who echoed it back to me.

"Like a Hot Girl Walk . . ." The crowd echoed again.

"Because a Hot Girl Walk don't stop!" We repeated the cheer a few times, and each time, I could feel everyone's walls coming down. Throughout the walk, people even started to cheer on their own.

Which leads me to the title of this section: breaking down walls starts with just one person. It can be nerve-wracking going to an event where you don't know anyone. Knowing this, I always do at least one thing to break the ice. People take cues from community leaders, and if a leader is nervous or only talking to their friends, everyone else will follow suit. The leader sets the tone for the community.

Whether you're looking to join or start a community, the greatest moment you have to look forward to is when those walls finally break down. It takes time for a community to evolve into a sisterhood, but the benefits are limitless. I've seen people support one another, create lasting friendships, or just offer an ear to listen during a challenging time. The feeling of belonging to a sisterhood is like knowing you have a net to catch you if you fall. It can empower you to take risks, try something new, or stand up for yourself if needed.

I had never felt such joy as I did that first time in Miami. It was a moment of pure sisterhood and community, of joy and camaraderie. But it was a moment created because of the people who showed up. I thought something like that would only happen once, so imagine my surprise when it happened again.

We hosted our first-ever Hot Girl Walk in the UK in 2023. I hadn't left the United States in over a decade, and it was my first time traveling abroad alone. I had expected to have some nerves, heading to a place where I didn't really know anyone. But instead, I felt peace. Even though I had never met the people attending, even though it was our first ever event in the UK, I already felt that sense of community.

Over 400 people showed up. Two women jumped in to help me pass out the bracelets and totes I brought. One woman saw that my suitcase (which held all the tote bags) was getting filled with rain, so she moved it under a covering. A few people even came up to tell me their friends or family had attended Hot Girl Walks in the States and how excited they were that we finally came to the UK. This is sisterhood. This is that feeling that you can't always see. This is the power of community.

Finding Community

If you're not ready to start and lead a community on your own, do some research into communities near you and join some of them. As I mentioned in the earlier exercise, you can find community at school, with people you work with, during activities, or through your hobbies. You'd be surprised how many groups are already out there, attempting to build strong communities with like-minded and diverse people. All it takes is one step. Commit yourself to attend each meeting. Take the time to get to know people there and build that trust. Soon enough, you'll start to feel the walls coming down.

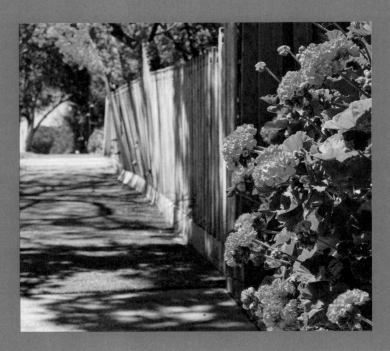

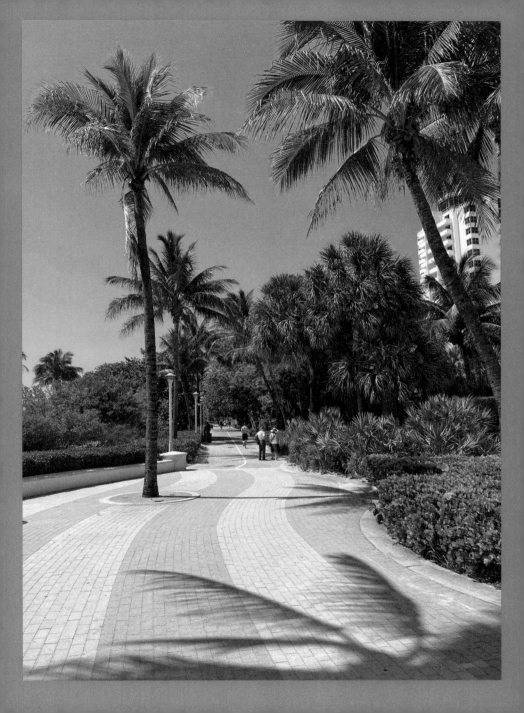

Inspired by
Giovanna's Story

One of my favorite parts of Hot Girl Walks is meeting people at all different stages of their journeys. Some may be starting a fitness journey; some have just come out on the other end of something; and some don't realize this walk is about to be the change they need. It's incredible to hear about so many different lives and paths, yet they've all found their place together on a Hot Girl Walk. Looking around at all the faces, each with a different story to tell and a lesson to learn, is a striking moment of "sonder." Sonder is the realization that everyone you see and meet has a life as complex as your own. You may have experienced sonder in a random conversation you had with someone in the airport. Then you walked around realizing all these people were headed around the world to hundreds of different locations and yet were here in the same place all at once. Or maybe it's a feeling you think about when you find your soulmate, whether platonic or romantic.

To exist is a miracle in itself. Regardless of your belief system, it's important to recognize the rarity of being put on this Earth. Then, to see this miracle multiplied exponentially, to realize that you are here with this group of people all at the same time but with different purposes. It can be overwhelming, but it's beautiful.

Giovanna summarizes this concept in a lovely way:

" My favorite Hot Girl Walk memory is the first one I attended in Los Angeles. It was also the very first day that I arrived in the city while traveling solo. I straight away felt a part of something, a community of people like me, of strong girls like me. I've met a lot of people who are still in my life and are supporting me in my current projects.

My best advice to give to someone starting on their Hot Girl Walk journey is to never think that you have arrived and experienced everything. Life is beautiful. I discovered this after a severe depression that made me feel drained and also dependent on others. This year, however, I decided for the first time, at thirty-six years old, to travel alone. I rediscovered my strength and will to live. Because there will always be something waiting to be experienced for the first time."

While traveling by herself from the UK, Giovanna found a Hot Girl Walk in Los Angeles, California. She didn't know anyone at first, but she was able to find people she connected with. She beautifully states that one should "never think you have arrived and experienced *everything*." This is similar to the sentiment of Greek philosopher Heraclitus, who said that like a flowing river, you never step into the same river twice. The water is always moving and flowing just as the world is always moving around us. Each day is a new experience, an experience that nobody has lived before you, and an experience you will never have again.

The concept of sonder always allows me to look at the world with a new perspective. Just as I am rare and experiencing life for the first time, so is the person Hot Girl Walk-ing next to me.

DAILY EMPOWERMENT PRACTICES

Morning Routines for **Success**

I used to *hate* waking up early. At my corporate tech job, I had a 7 a.m. meeting to start every day. Whether I went to sleep at 10 p.m. or midnight, I would roll out of bed at 6:59 a.m. and open my laptop. I had always associated waking up early with being productive. As a type A person, productivity is my trigger word. However, it felt like so much pressure to be "productive." What does that even mean? To me, being productive requires getting every second of sleep before sitting in front of my laptop until 5 p.m.

This routine made life tough. I would wake up for work, feel exhausted once the day was over, and then go to sleep, with the only thing to look forward to being the weekend.

I fell into this routine for years. Until one day when I realized that I had free will, and I chose to make it my mission to reclaim my mornings. The first obstacle I had to overcome was feeling like my job was my purpose—which was essentially true, as it was the reason I was waking up every morning. Podcasters and wellness experts will tell you to get sunlight first thing in the morning, take a long walk, do a fasted workout, don't drink coffee until you've been up for two hours, and finish your morning with an ice-cold shower. While all these things are probably great for you, they didn't exactly sound better than the extra two hours of sleep I could be getting.

Instead, I started setting my alarm twenty minutes earlier to do *my* favorite thing: scroll on my phone. No, that isn't something wellness experts would recommend, but it did give me some precious me time before a long day of work. Those twenty minutes soon turned into an hour, until it became my favorite part of the day. Before long, I was adding 4-mile Hot Girl Walks to my morning routine. The morning became the one time of day when I wasn't getting bombarded by emails, and when I could listen to my favorite music or podcasts and even have time to scroll social media. I found myself going to sleep excited about the Hot Girl Walk and coffee I had planned the next day. Today, I have mastered my morning coffee recipe with the perfect amount of milk and vanilla syrup. Things like my daily coffee, Hot Girl Walks, and my self-care routine became anchors. They brought excitement and personality to my routine.

Now I go into my workday energized, and I'm someone who used to *never* claim to be a morning person. If you struggle with having a good morning routine, the question you need to ask yourself is, *Why do we save our favorite things to do until after work?* The best morning routine does not *need* to be productive, but it should set the tone for the rest of your day. We don't wake up to work; we wake up to live.

I think of my morning as a warm-up before a workout. Take the time to get your body ready for the workout, but don't push yourself so hard that you're too tired for the workout itself. Stretch and warm the muscles that you are going to use during the day. That way you can avoid pulling muscles or using poor posture because you prepared your mind and body for what was to come.

This is the only requirement that you should start implementing into your morning routine: warm-up. Some people find this solace in journaling, meditating, working out, having a nourishing breakfast, or even doing all these things. Just make sure to keep the weight of your morning routine low. Similar to when in the gym, low weight allows for a high amount of repetition. No matter what happens in life, the sun always rises, and you want your morning routine to repeat. If it's too hard, you'll be less likely to want to do it again the next day. Especially if it's new for you, the low weight is also low pressure. This warm-up is supposed to be something that makes you excited to wake up the next morning, not intimidated by it.

When I hear "morning routine," I think of the internet-famous "CEO morning routines," which tell tales of CEOs waking up at 3 a.m. to run 8 miles, do a cold plunge, sauna, cold shower, meditation, and eat an entire steak, all before they attend their first meeting at 8 a.m. If this is your speed, more power to you, but to me, this is unsustainable. The key here is that a healthy lifestyle is defined by sustainability, not intensity.

Evening Reflections

What you do in your evening is the shadow of how you live during the day. What you do at night is more important than what you do during the day. The thoughts that you think when you close your eyes in bed are your truest thoughts and feelings, representing who you are as a person and what you desire in life.

A successful evening routine should allow you to (1) continue the discipline that you have formed in yourself during the day, (2) fully unwind from your day, and (3) prepare you to have another successful day tomorrow. Let's discuss these pillars.

Discipline

When the sun goes down, it's tempting to write off your day completely, however, this isn't the time to give up on yourself. As we discussed in the self-appreciation chapter (page 56), confidence comes from trust in yourself that you will follow through on what you say you are going to do.

I love working out to end my day, especially after working from home, because it gives me time to delineate my work life from my home life. Whatever happens during my day, I leave it at the door of my workout. The goal for me is to burn off any excess negative energy that I've accumulated during the day. This can be done in the form of a Hot Girl Walk, a gym session, a workout class, etc. To take it even further, I love to give myself a personal challenge within that workout to make it fun and motivating. Showing discipline for yourself is a form of self-care. Here are some examples:

★ **Take up a personal project.** Personal projects that are separate from work are important in keeping your identity more complex than just your job. There are more facets to you than your profession. Personal projects can look like: hosting a book club, writing a book, coordinating a party, planning a wedding, etc. These projects all lead to bigger goals and should fulfill your other interests. The challenge with a personal project is that it takes discipline to cross the finish line. Any project has its own struggles, but there is compartmentalization that comes with working on a project outside of work or school. Do something that allows you to break away from the thinking that you normally have to do at work or school or that exercises the parts of your brain that you may want to use later on in your career. On the other hand, a project can always be used as a side hustle or as currency when applying to new jobs. It shows employers that you have a life and interests outside of work and that you have the drive to complete something of your own.

★ **Live a healthier lifestyle.** Being healthy isn't always the easy choice, because if it were, everyone would be healthy all the time. "Healthy" can mean different things to different people, but overall, it typically includes eating more whole foods, working out, and cooking at home. Most of us are lucky to have convenience at our fingertips when it comes to food. So, sometimes the easy choice to swing by a fast-food place or order your favorite burrito is hard to avoid. It is harder to think of what you want to cook, go to the grocery store, and walk past all the temptations along the way. But there are tricks you can use to ease the process, like prepping meals for the week or booking workout classes, which have strict cancellation policies, ahead of time. At the end of the day, we have tens of thousands of choices we have to make, and it takes discipline to choose the hard option. Remember that this discipline is a service to yourself and, again, a form of self-care. You're fulfilling your promise to yourself to live a healthier lifestyle that the future you will benefit from.

★ **Attend social outings.** Depending on your introversion or extroversion, socializing could be self-care or something you force yourself to do. When life gets busy, seeing your friends or acquaintances may be the last thing on your mind. But having a social life should be a priority if it isn't already. As an introverted-extrovert myself, I often have to force myself out of the house to go on a social outing, but afterwards, I feel fulfilled every time. If you are not going out to see friends at least once a week, challenge yourself to say yes more. Making time to fill your social wells is a discipline that will help combat any future loneliness.

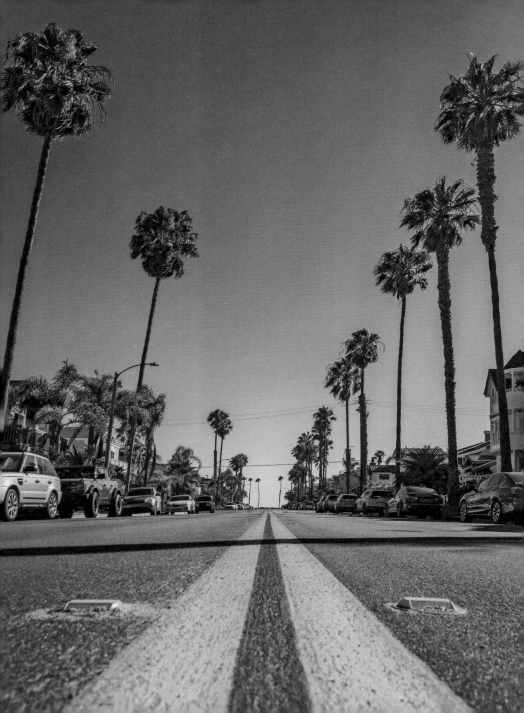

There are only so many hours in the evening, so the way you honor the pillars of discipline may look different each night. The idea here is to honor them in some way, even if you've had a long and trying day. Practicing discipline is a form of self-care, even on the days when it doesn't feel fun.

Reset

Once you have eaten dinner, gone to the gym, and worked on your project, it is time to reset your space. Every evening, I clean my kitchen, do the dishes, and get my room in the best shape it can be as a gift to my morning self. Ending and beginning the day in a clean space is as much of a mental gift to yourself as it is a visual gift. I wholeheartedly agree with the idea that clear spaces equal a clear mind.

The process of resetting your space can be meditative as well, as it involves somewhat mindless tasks. They can be done by yourself, becoming valuable, quality time to reflect on your day. Or even better, they can be done with your roommate or partner. With a significant other, doing chores together helps reinforce the idea that you're a team. It's a time that is both productive and necessary.

If you have trouble motivating yourself to get your cleaning done, I recommend setting a twenty-minute timer. This allows your brain to block out anything else that you may need to accomplish and focus on the task at hand. Do as much as you can within those twenty minutes. At the end of the week, you'll have much less cleaning to worry about.

Self-Care

This is the portion of your evening routine when it is truly time to unwind. The definition of self-care in this pillar is something you *want* to do—even though this could be a need, self-care should primarily be a want.

My ultimate self-care routine includes a nice long shower utilizing all my favorite scented body wash and lotions, eating a nourishing dinner, and curling up to watch my favorite TV show. I do this nearly every single night, and it never gets old. My friend used to say that I am not "high maintenance," but I am "high frequency," meaning it doesn't take a lot to make me happy, but I like to be happy all the time. To do this, I nourish myself with little luxuries, like a lotion that has a scent attached to a good memory, making my space feel special with a lit candle, and making my night as dreamy as possible. These little moments of indulgence are the things I look forward to every night and that bring me joy without being a financial or physical burden.

When I graduated from college and started my full-time job, I felt like I only had two days to unwind and have fun before having to go right back to it on Monday. It felt like a repetitive and never-ending cycle. I knew this wasn't healthy, and my main problem was I didn't have any source of enjoyment during the week. I even fell off my daily Hot Girl Walks and my mental health was worse than ever. So, the first change I made was to reimplement my daily walks, which allowed me to create a distinction between work and relaxing during the week. After working up a sweat, I'd take my evening shower.

Self-care should be something that makes a part of your day a bit more special than it would normally be. It may be something as small as making the effort to put your towel in the dryer before your shower so you can wrap yourself in warmth, reading a book, or doing a small craft. Before moving on to the next section, take note of five little luxuries you can implement into your evening routine. What classifies self-care for you?

Reflect

The final pillar of a "perfect" evening routine is reflection. Keep a journal next to your bed and take five minutes to write down how you felt today, what you did, what you're proud of yourself for, and what you're grateful for. Save your goal setting for your morning Hot Girl Walk; this is your time to go to bed with the most positive state of mind.

You'll see it written in every self-care book and hear it on every self-improvement podcast: you should start journaling. I'm here to confirm that I subscribe to the practice. When life becomes chaotic, or your thoughts are a bit too loud for your mind, taking the time to write it out on paper—to dump your thoughts, in a coherent train of thought or not—provides a moment of relief unlike anything else.

Now's the time to get a journal and start writing out everything in your brain. Journaling gives your mind room to rest and make space for tomorrow's thoughts. You can use this journal to look back and reflect, or throw it away once it's full. Use it however works best for you. I promise you'll thank me.

The purpose of these methodologies isn't to overwhelm you. Use them like ingredients in a recipe—pick and choose which ones you want to use more or less of. Because everyone is different, finding the balance that works best for you will take some trial and error. Start by measuring with your heart, as your intuition usually knows best. These pillars can also be something you spread across your week to fit into your schedule. Again, it isn't always attainable for everyone to be able to implement all these pillars in one day. If you can hit them all throughout the week, that's still an accomplishment. These are the methods that I've found on my journey, but it's up to you to make them work for you and your life.

Learn to Love Repetition

Making your daily routine special keeps it desirable. It took me a long time to get settled in the repetition. If you find yourself living for the weekend, it is because you are not happy with your routine. Remember that you are in control of what your day looks like. These pillars of morning and evening routines are a balancing act of your wants and needs.

Growing up in dance classes, repetition formed the basic structure of everything we did. The same songs playing on repeat, often practicing the same movements, focusing on small adjustments to make the big picture look right. What I learned from this process was how to find beauty and something "new" in the repetition. Like listening to a song on repeat, reading a book again, watching a movie multiple times, or even learning the routines in relationships. We can find something new and fresh, without changing anything about the object, if we let our perspective change.

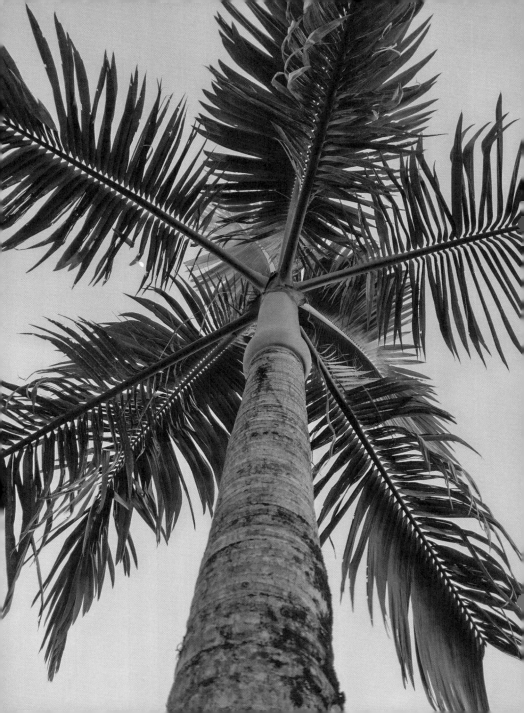

Inspired by
Anaisse's Story

There's immense strength in repetition. Walking is a repetitive motion. Right, left, right, left. One foot after the other. It's predictable and reliable, which is where it derives its strength. I always find that walking puts me into a "flow state." A flow state is that feeling when you're doing a task and, colloquially speaking, "in the zone." A flow state feels great because you're able to effortlessly complete a task. There is, however, a set of conditions that allows for a flow state: it must be challenging but not frustratingly so; it has a clear goal; you feel a sense of concentration and control; and it becomes intrinsically rewarding.

Hot Girl Walk-ing is the perfect way to put me into a flow state. After my walks, I find that my brain is clear, and I'm prepared to attack whatever task lies ahead of me.

Anaisse recognizes a similar feeling of strength on her Hot Girl Walks:

> 66 **Hot Girl Walks make me feel empowered and strong! They're a great way to reconnect with my mind and body when I'm stressed with life. This community shows me that women around the world are so connected for a cause to better themselves. It gives me hope that this next generation is strong!**

My best advice to give someone starting their Hot Girl Walk journey is to do whatever you want. Show others that you're strong and you run the show."

Repetitive tasks like walking allow your mind to focus. What may have been stressing you out suddenly becomes clear. When I am stressed, I manifest it as tension in my body. My sympathetic nervous system (the one that controls your fight-or-flight response) is firing, making my heart race and my thoughts run quickly. I clench my jaw and tense my shoulders. By Hot Girl Walk-ing, I'm redirecting my body's sympathetic response to the activity of walking; meanwhile, I'm able to get back in touch with my mind.

Anaisse felt a similar connection between mind and body on her Hot Girl Walks. Pairing the positive effects of the Hot Girl Walk with the benefits of having a community, Anaisse even cited feelings of hope after meeting fellow Hot Girl Walk-ers who all believed in the positive message of the movement.

Finding strength in our footsteps gives us power and shows us that there will always be another step to take. It settles our mind by just putting one foot after the other. It's small changes like these that lead to big ones.

A POCKETFUL OF INSPIRATION

125

PORTABLE
PRACTICES *FOR*
Busy Lives

132

STAY *INSPIRED*
ON THE **Move**

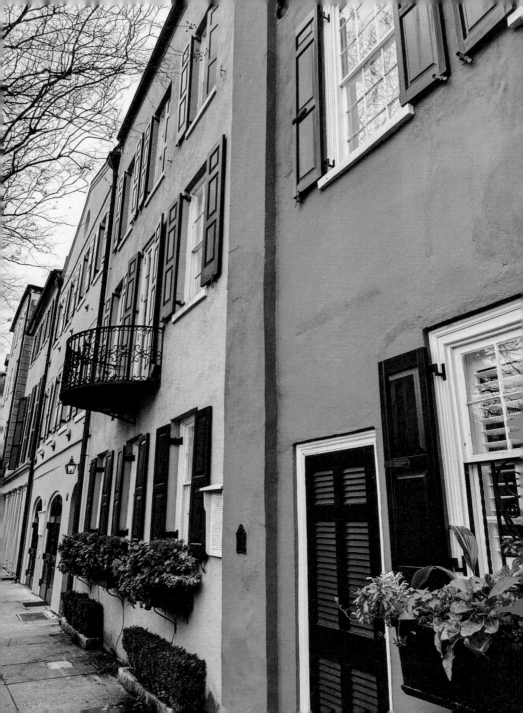

Portable *Practices* *for* Busy Lives

By now, you should realize that wellness is not defined by green juices and expensive massages. Wellness is innate to humans. Oftentimes, we just need to reconnect with what our bodies need and want and pull our focus away from technology and toward the world around us.

Gratitude practice and visualization are not new concepts. With growing research on these topics, we can understand why they repeatedly return to the zeitgeist: because they work. Many studies suggest the secret to living a long life is community and connection. Resisting gratitude, lacking self-appreciation, and living too solitary of a life does not produce success. It is only through a combination of these things that a busy person can find fulfillment and maintain it for a long time to come.

The methodology of the Hot Girl Walk is a cumulation of these techniques and how I adapted them to make sense for my lifestyle and my state of mind. These techniques are meant to be adaptable to any and every lifestyle and should be inclusive and accessible to all. In the first TikTok I made, where I shared the Hot Girl Walk, I said that the most important part of the walk is taking that energy and carrying it with you throughout the entire day. So, with that in mind, here are some scenarios and portable practices to help you carry your Hot Girl Walk energy with you no matter where you are or what you're doing.

Managing Anxiety

Imagine this: It's five minutes before you're about to give the biggest presentation of your career—or maybe a big speech for class, a performance, or an interview. There isn't time to take a 4-mile walk, but you need to quell your nerves and maybe some of that imposter syndrome that has begun to kick in. In situations like this, where you only have five minutes or less, there's no time to confront your feelings; you just need to put your state of mind in the right place to complete your task successfully.

Four Powerful Words

Squeeze your fists together as hard as you can for thirty seconds and say the following four words: *dare to be great*.

It can almost feel more comfortable to give in to your anxiety, but you shouldn't let your anxiety get the best of you in an important moment like this. While it is scary to go out there and leave it all on the floor, if you take that leap to be your very best, you'll be more satisfied with the outcome than if you let your anxieties take over. You have prepared for this moment. The only way to fail is to *let* yourself fail. Take five minutes and make them count.

Making a Mistake

Unfortunately, mistakes happen all the time—at work, school, and in life. Sometimes they are small, and you can get away with them; other times, your boss puts a ten minute check-in on your calendar, you embarrass yourself in front of a client, or you forget your paper was due today, not next week.

As a perfectionist, making mistakes are devastating to me. Big or small, they chip away at my self-image. They affirm every terrible thought I have about myself. Every second of empowerment I've accumulated and every affirmation I've learned pales in comparison to the negative thoughts that overtake my brain. The most important thing to do at this moment is stop the singular mistake from spreading. What's done is done, but there is still a chance that you can save everything else around it before the fire spreads. Mistakes usually have a domino effect when we allow them to overwhelm us. They can make us flustered and then we do things that we would not normally do.

I like to use a visualization technique to compartmentalize the mistake rather than let it universalize in my mind.

File it Away

Use the following to visualize how you can keep a mistake as one singular moment and not let it turn into something more disastrous.

Picture your brain with infinite cabinets and drawers that are full of every single action you've ever made. Each action is sorted into sections defined by your personality traits. These sections are your identity. For example, I identify as a reliable person, so each time I do something reliable, it gets filed into my "reliable" section, and the section grows and grows as I keep adding currency. When I make a mistake at work, it doesn't take away from all the millions of times I was a reliable person; it just gets added into my "mistakes" section, which doesn't hinder how reliable I already am. With this visualization, watch your mistake get placed in its own cabinet, and let it be filed away next to the millions of cabinets that make up your personality.

By doing this, you can start to mentally come to terms with your mistake. You can't undo your mistakes; the only choice is to be accountable and move forward. If your boss wants to talk to you about it, denying or making excuses will only make it worse. With confidence of your typical reliability, you can assure your boss that it won't happen again. Soon, you'll be able to move on with the rest of your day without letting the weight of this mistake weigh you down.

Taking a Leap

Nobody ever did anything great without first doing something scary. When I was deciding between staying at my corporate job or leaving to pursue my own business, it took many months of deliberation. The choice was obvious in my gut, but it was made complicated by fears of giving up a stable salary, upcoming commission checks, and a great health insurance policy, that muddied a decision that was otherwise clear. It made the decision extremely challenging.

I am infamously indecisive. It's not the idea of making the decision that is challenging to me, but the permanence of leaving the alternative behind. Life is just a great big wheel of decisions. We are constantly choosing one path over the other, but there are some choices that feel too big to make quickly. Especially without knowing if it is the right choice or if there will be an option to go back once you've chosen. But that's a spiral that we know to avoid, so we're not going to carry on down that road again.

The exercise I use involves a pros and cons list. When dealing with big decisions, get the people around you involved. Talk to everyone you know and get their opinion. You want to weigh every single outcome. Having multiple people hear your dilemma and give their perspective on the situation will make the choice much clearer than if you only have your thoughts on it. At this point, you *know* what the right decision is; you just need the courage to charge ahead.

Repeat After Me

"Whatever I choose to do, it will be a success.
The only failure is to give up on myself."

Dealing with Rejection

Putting yourself out there only to be rejected can be demoralizing. Especially if you haven't just been rejected one time but time after time after time. Some people let this fear of rejection hold them back from putting themselves out there in the first place. In this scenario, however, you've put yourself out there, maybe several times, and have been rejected once again.

I've been rejected more times than I can count in many different areas of my life: personal, professional, and social. But at this point, rejection motivates me. I still get that sinking feeling when I initially receive a rejection, but within moments it washes away. More times than not, rejection has nothing to do with you on a personal level but stems from elements out of your control. If we let rejection get the best of us, it can manifest itself into a self-fulfilling prophecy where we reject ourselves before we can be rejected.

Instead, think of it this way: If you're doing your best to be your best, a rejection is just one step closer to an acceptance. Like making a mistake, rejections can challenge your identity and make you doubt yourself, but I've found a few affirmations that help instead of letting feelings of rejection keep me down:

"Each rejection means I'm one step closer to success."

"This rejection has nothing to do with my abilities."

"I am worthy of every opportunity."

"Pushing through rejection makes me stronger."

With these quick empowerment techniques to deal with rejection, one day you'll be invincible. This attitude will help propel you to reach beyond your perceived limits, and you may even surprise yourself.

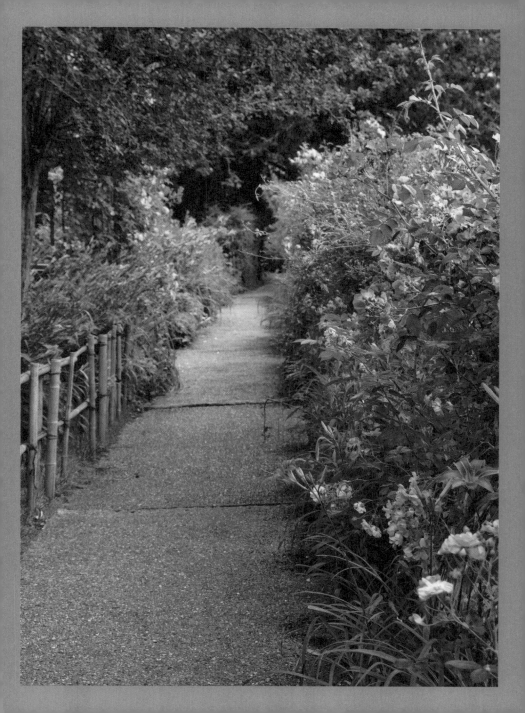

Stay *Inspired* on *the* Move

Motivation does not exist. That's all you need to know when you want to change your life. We make lofty goals with expectations that every day is going to be like New Year's Day. We create big plans to go to the gym and live off only salads, but the motivation quickly fades as each day passes. As we've discussed in past chapters, it's best to start with smaller, more manageable goals, and make changes in your habits one step at a time.

Though motivation does not exist, we can manufacture it. Motivation doesn't just fall into your lap and suddenly light you up, especially after a long day or week. The best strategy for getting out of a rut—when you feel like you don't have the energy or the spirit to do absolutely anything—is to start small. Tell yourself, "I'm going to set a two-minute timer and clean my room for just those two minutes." Without any pressure to go beyond those two minutes, you're likely to clean for two minutes, then throw a load of laundry in, make your bed, and go work out. Before you know it, those two minutes have turned into ten. It's a domino effect that starts with one small action.

This is why I love Hot Girl Walks. A Hot Girl Walk can be just ten minutes walking around my neighborhood or up the block. It is a low-commitment activity that I have a hard time finding an excuse not to do.

Short Hot Girl Walks after work always help me shift my thoughts from exhaustion to excitement. A Hot Girl Walk of just thirty minutes can be all it takes to shut off your thoughts from work and give yourself some well-deserved me time. I don't feel any pressure to go on a Hot Girl Walk, hoping I'll suddenly have a burst of energy and exercise afterward or do much-needed chores or cook dinner, but the formula of pop music and walking endorphins gives me a much-needed boost that I would have never gotten had I just decided to nap straight after work.

Now my brain associates my Hot Girl Walks with productivity. It's almost as if I've conditioned myself to queue motivation afterward. Contrary to the fallacy that it will carry you through life, motivation is a conscious decision you have to make. I now know the formula needed to kick-start my motivation; it's just about getting up and doing it.

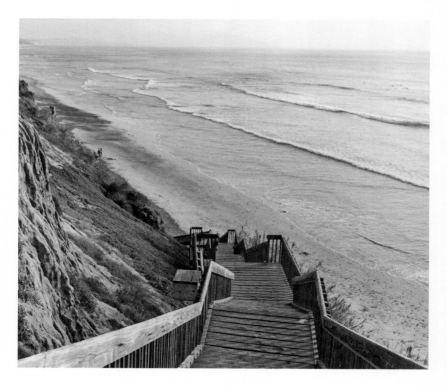

Inspired by
Sabrina's
Story

Hot Girl Walks seem so simple at face value: go outside, take a walk, and think about gratitude, goals, and how hot (confident) you are. Its simplicity is appealing. "Easy enough," you might think, but the lessons learned are limitless.

Sabrina from New York recognizes that a Hot Girl Walk isn't *just* a walk:

    66 **I Hot Girl Walk because it's my time to clear my head, boost my confidence, and just focus on myself. It's not just about getting some steps in—it's about feeling good, looking good, and reminding myself that I'm *that* girl.**

Hot Girl Walks have honestly changed my life. At first, I just started doing them to clear my head and get some fresh air, but now they're my favorite part of the day. It's my time to focus on myself, listen to good music or a podcast, and just vibe. Mentally, I feel so much more confident and less stressed. They're like my little reset button whenever I'm feeling off. Physically, I have more energy, and I've even noticed my mood is way better. Plus, they give me time to think about my goals and hype myself up. It's not just about walking—it's about

feeling good, looking good, and knowing I'm doing something positive for myself. Honestly, 10/10 recommend!

Hot Girl Walks are more than just steps—they're self-care in motion. Stay consistent, layer up in winter, and let every walk remind you of your strength and confidence. Keep moving, keep glowing!"

What started as a small practice for Sabrina turned into a cornerstone of her routine. Self-care can be more than just lounging around and staying inside. Hot Girl Walks are universally beneficial, tackling a myriad of corners in your life. Movement is a form of self-care, but it can also be a medium for meditation. You just have to start.

YOUR EMPOWERMENT TOOLKIT

149

ENCOURAGEMENT
FOR THE JOURNEY
Ahead

150

RECOMMENDED
Reading

153

Resources

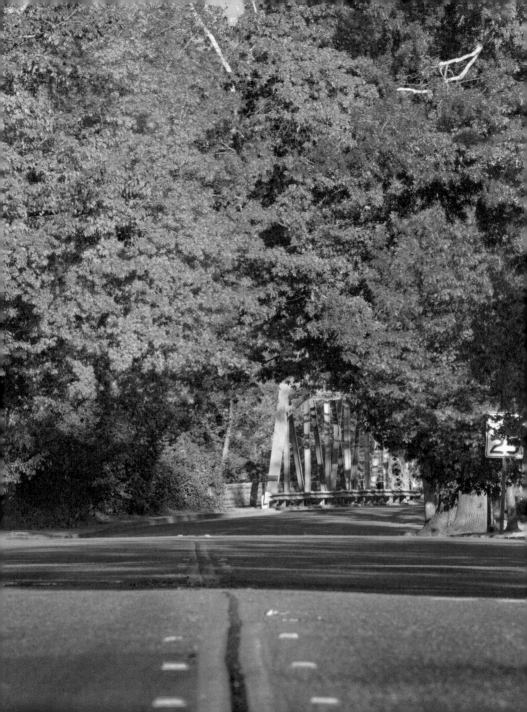

Congratulations! You made it to the end of the book. That was a lot of information, so I hope you have highlighted, tabbed, or taken notes to look back on. Below is a quick wrap-up of the main ideas and tools we discussed in the book to help jog your memory whenever you need a refresher about the Hot Girl Walk movement.

Cultivating Gratitude

PAGE 22

⭐ **Gratitude is the secret to everything!** Gratitude is our biggest hack to happiness, built into our brains as a natural reward system.

⭐ **We are in control of our happiness.** More than you'd probably think. Take control of your happiness, starting with gratitude practice.

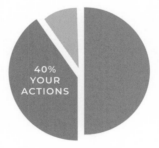

⭐ **Practicing gratitude is not complicated.** It's as simple as saying "thank you" to the things we take for granted. Start small by thanking your ability to indulge in a simple pleasure like going on a walk to being grateful for your family and friends. Feel free to share this grateful feeling with those around you and make the words *thank you* a large part of your vocabulary.

Setting and Achieving Goals

PAGE 36

★ **Hot Girl Walk *As If . . .*** you have already reached your goals, whatever they may be. This is a scenario-based method where you convince yourself that in any given scenario, you've already walked away with a win. It's about starting with a confident mindset so that you handle the situation with confidence.

★ **Discover your best self.** Use your Hot Girl Walks to literally walk a mile in the shoes of the "best version" of you. Be specific about who the best version of you is so that you can fully embody them.

★ **Make SMART goals.** These are meant to guide you in creating achievable and specific goals to reach your "best self." With actionable steps and goalposts to keep you on track to success, you will reach your best self in no time.

★ **Create and break habits.** Habits are the steps taken to reach the finish line. These habits are the activities you do every day without having to think about them. If we can change our bad habits into good ones, we can use them to our advantage to make long-term lifestyle changes, ultimately helping us to reach our goals.

★ **Motivation is fleeting!** Habits are the life vests that keep you afloat when your motivation only appears a few days a month (if you're lucky).

★ **Do the impossible.** Challenge yourself to do a task you've deemed "impossible," starting once every other month and building up to do it weekly. The purpose is to show yourself that you can surprise yourself. You can do anything you set your mind to.

A few methods to create habits are:

1 **Habit stacking:** Place your desired habit on top of your current habit instead of trying to quit cold turkey.

2 **Temptation bundling:** Wrap up your desired habit with an action you *want*.

3 **Make it easy:** Make your desired habit an easy choice. Remove all barriers between yourself and achieving this habit.

4 **Identify:** Make your new habit a part of your identity. Remove the imposter syndrome and embody the person you want to be when you perform your new habit.

Embracing Self-Appreciation

PAGE 56

★ **Confidence may not come naturally.** In a world where comparison has become the norm, it's hard to appreciate our own self-worth. I realized I had to train myself to be confident and found strategies that helped use the "fake it till you make it mindset" to bring out my true confidence and feelings about myself.

★ **Find your glow:** Take note of the traits that make you unique. Focus on building confidence in these traits, as they're formative to your identity. Confidence in your core traits builds universal confidence and can help you begin to find your inner glow.

★ Sticky notes of power: Use sticky notes as visual reminders of your traits that make you powerful. Every week, take time to nurse these traits, growing in strength and confidence.

★ HIIT Confidence Practice: Challenge yourself to have ten minutes of unbridled confidence. Take note of what it feels like when you wear confidence on your skin. Challenge yourself to leave out feelings of doubt, and even let these feelings linger beyond the ten-minute exercise. Most of the time, all we ever need is about ten minutes of confidence, whether it's a job interview, presentation, or a first date. It just takes ten minutes to show up as 100 percent of you.

Building Resilience

PAGE 72

★ What does confidence mean? Confidence does not mean you never face doubts or challenges, and it doesn't mean life becomes easier; you just get stronger.

★ Overcoming the tornado of negativity: A negative spiral occurs when your emotions for a specific circumstance are disproportionate to the circumstance itself. We used a tornado to help visualize the nosedive our thoughts can take when we let negativity overpower us. Being alone with your thoughts allows negative thoughts to take space, but learning to stop the cycle of negativity is essential to building resilience.

★ Personify your negative thoughts: Imagining your negative thoughts coming from a voice outside yourself helps you to better understand what these thoughts are trying to communicate to you. Most of the time, you are your own biggest critic, and your thoughts are meant to save you from disappointment if things don't work out. When these thoughts are personified, we can understand and honor them to the degree that they should (or should not) be honored.

★ **Confront your inner voice:** To that negative inner voice, say, "Thank you for letting me know. I know you have my best interests at heart but dwelling on the negative won't bring a positive."

★ **Law of Attraction:** The Law of Attraction is the principle that positive thoughts breed positive results, and vice versa for negative thoughts.

★ **Manage negative thoughts:** Learn not to let negativity get the best of you; it can have power in your life if you let it. We shouldn't let these negative thoughts influence outcomes in our lives.

The Pull Back, Look In Method:

Pull Back: Imagine yourself soaring outside your body and take a third-person perspective of the scenario. In other words, remove yourself from your emotions and look at the situation objectively or professionally.

Look In: Now that you have an unbiased, omniscient view of your situation, you should be able to understand what happened, what is going on, and what the next steps are.

When things happen outside of your control, it may be jarring and spur you to act immediately. This exercise forces us to look outside of our circumstances. Hot Girl Walks are *essential* to the Pull Back, Look In approach. When you are at work or school and surrounded by negative thoughts, they can seem all-consuming. Taking a step back forces you into a new perspective. You realize that the world is still turning. Let this new perspective soothe you and keep you from falling into that negative spiral.

Embracing Sisterhood

PAGE 85

★ **What is sisterhood?** Sisterhood, next to community, is the final secret to a fulfilling and happy life. Sisterhood can come in many forms, including your family or relationships that are forged outside of blood. Sisterhood can also exist in groups that share a goal and a journey. Sisterhood, no matter what form it may take, is valuable.

★ **Make a commitment:** Commitment is the difference between showing up or staying at home, going up to someone new or keeping to yourself, and congratulating someone or staying silent. Commitment builds trust.

★ **Spend time, earn trust:** It takes time to build a community into a sisterhood. By continuously showing up for one another, time and time again, this trust can be built.

★ **Break down walls:** To build trust, you must help bring down the walls we have as people. Yes, this can take time, but as a community leader, you can use your role to lead by example.

Daily Empowerment Practices

PAGE 106

★ **Why are routines important?** Morning and evening routines help set structure to keep empowerment as a common thread in your life.

★ **Morning routine:** Your morning routine is your warm-up. It shouldn't be daunting or challenging. It should be something that makes you excited when you go to bed and excited when you wake up in the morning. It should also be sustainable. No matter what happens in life, the sun always rises, and your morning routine must repeat. Especially if a morning routine is new for you, an easier routine creates less pressure to succeed, making it more likely that you'll wake up to do it again. A healthy lifestyle is defined by sustainability, not intensity.

★ **Evening Routine:** What you do in your evening is the shadow of how you live during the day. The thoughts you think when you close your eyes are your truest reflections of who you are and what you desire. There are multiple pillars to a "successful" evening routine. It allows you to maintain discipline, unwind, and prepare for another productive day. Use each method like ingredients in a recipe—you can adjust as needed. They can also be spread across your week to fit your schedule. You control what your routine looks like. These pillars are a balance of your wants and needs.

★ **Discipline:** Confidence comes from trust in yourself that you will follow through on what you promise yourself. Stretching your discipline into the evening solidifies those thoughts in your head that you follow through on your word and have the ability to do what needs to be done. You can go to sleep and be satisfied with yourself. In the chapter, I give examples of how discipline can be exercised in your nightly routine, knowing that each evening may look a little different. Discipline can be personal projects, healthier lifestyle choices, or social outings.

★ **Reset:** Once you have eaten dinner, gone to the gym, and worked on your project, it is time to reset your space. Clear spaces help clear your mind.

★ **Self-Care:** This is the portion of your evening routine when it is truly time to unwind. The definition of self-care in this pillar is something you "want" to do; it could be a need, but it is primarily a want. Take a nice long shower, draw up a bath, put on a sheet mask, turn on your guilty pleasure TV show. Whatever fills your cup, allow it to fill space in your evening routine. Take note of "little luxuries," i.e, small indulgences you can implement to make your evenings feel special and therefore exciting to replicate.

★ **Reflect:** Keep a journal next to your bed and allow yourself five minutes to write down how the day made you feel, what you did, what you're proud of yourself for, and what you're grateful for. Save your goal setting for your morning Hot Girl Walk; this is your time to go to bed with the most positive state of mind.

Next Steps

I implore you to go on a Hot Girl Walk if you haven't already. After reading this book, you know the steps to take on your walk. But most importantly, think of the things you're grateful for, your goals, and how HOT you are. I've given you a lot of tools and methodologies to help empower you to be your best self. Use one tool or use them all. It starts with just one step. You'll know what to do for the next one.

A Pocketful of Inspiration

PAGE 122

✴ **Sustain the energy of a Hot Girl Walk.** The most important part of the Hot Girl Walk is to take that Hot Girl energy and carry it with you throughout the entire day. So, with that in mind, there are portable practices to help you keep your Hot Girl Walk energy all day, no matter where you are or what you're doing.

✴ **Four powerful words.** When dealing with anxiety, clench your hands into tight fists and say, "Dare to be great."

✴ **File it away.** When you've made a mistake, visualize the room of your personality divided into cabinets. Remember that a mistake does not hinder other parts of your personality, such as how reliable you are.

✴ **Make a pros and cons list.** Before taking a leap, ask the people around you to give their opinion so that you have weighed every possible outcome and feel confident in your decision.

✴ **Counteract the feelings of rejection.** To help deal with rejection, digest the news as empowerment. Think of each rejection as one step closer to your goal than you were before.

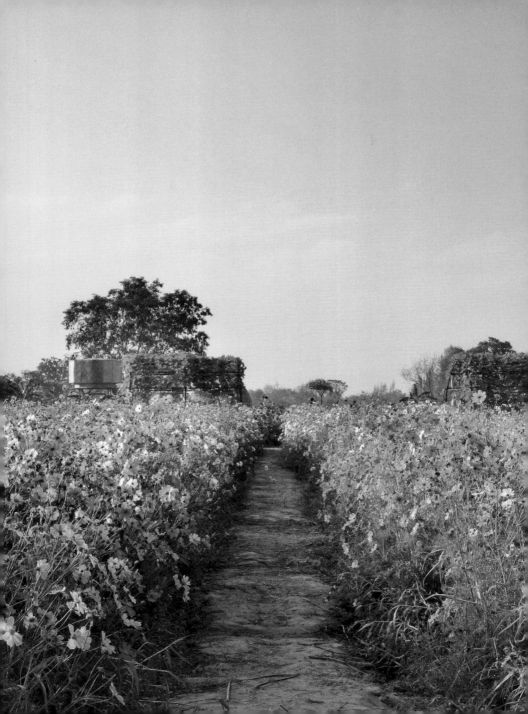

Encouragement for the Journey Ahead

You are stronger and more powerful than you give yourself credit for. I hope you use these techniques to empower you to achieve not just one of your goals but your mind's wildest dreams. By now, you should understand the power you have radiating inside of you, waiting for you to take it and run with it.

As a final thought, I'll share with you the thought experiment I do annually. It's the one that changed my life:

> Imagine it's the end of your life. You have the opportunity to meet with someone to review every single moment of your life. In front of you, they place a sheet of paper with every goal/hope/dream you have ever had. Then they look at you and say: "You had the tools to make all these things come true. Why didn't you make it happen?"

Your dreams are not so far out of reach as you might think they are. You have everything you need to make your dreams a reality, *so what is holding you back?*

With that thought in mind, let yourself be free of obstacles. You know you have the power to overcome challenges and get to the finish line. Take this energy and carry it with you every day. That is what being a Hot Girl is all about. It's not about looking a certain way or fitting in a box; it is about letting your inner glow shine.

All you ever need to remember is gratitude, goals, and confidence.

Recommended
Reading

When I was offered the chance to create this book, there were a few books that I had read and loved and knew I wanted to mimic or at least shout-out, as they helped me get to the place I am today. If, after reading this, you're looking for your next book, these are the ones I highly recommend and why.

Start with Why by Simon Sinek

When it comes to goal setting, having a strong sense of "why" is important in anchoring us. As we learned throughout this book, motivation is fleeting. Sinek shares stories of inspirational leaders throughout history and the one thing they all have in common: "why." If you're starting a journey to better yourself in some way, start with this book, and, as the title says, *Start with Why*.

The Defining Decade: Why Your Twenties Matter—And How to Make the Most of Them Now by Meg Jay

Meg Jay is a psychologist who works specifically with clients in their twenties. She shares their stories and what they've learned during this pivotal decade. This is the book I send to all my friends in their twenties—if they haven't read it already. In the age of social media and comparison culture, it's a good reminder that, *no*, not everyone has it "all figured out," and you don't need to have it figured out either.

Flow: The Psychology of Optimal Experience by Mihaly Csikszentmihalyi

Finding flow in everyday life is a key to cultivating happiness. It's all about finding enjoyment and creativity on a daily basis. Csikszentmihalyi teaches you how to harness this state to find happiness in life. I like to think of flow as another life hack. I use many of the concepts from his book on my daily Hot Girl Walks to enter a state of flow and sustain it throughout my day.

Atomic Habits by James Clear

If you're interested in learning more about creating long-lasting changes in your life, this book is the one to read. It's digestible and easy to implement the practices in your life. Many of its principles have been life-changing as I've had more and more responsibilities and less and less time.

Awe: The New Science of Everyday Wonder and How it Can Transform Your Life by Dacher Keltner

Dacher Keltner is a professor at UC Berkeley and a faculty member at the Greater Good Science Center. The Greater Good Science Center is where I had the privilege to take the class "Science of Happiness," which taught me that happiness is accessible to everyone and explained gratitude's role in happiness.

In this book, Keltner explores feelings of awe and its importance. He doesn't say it in his book, but awe is a great tool to use on your next Hot Girl Walk.

The Greater Good Science Center has many articles and resources on happiness. There is so much incredible research on this topic that the GGSC has completed and compiled. I implore you to look at their website: https://ggsc.berkeley.edu/.

The Gratitude Project: How the Science of Thankfulness Can Rewire Our Brains for Resilience, Optimism, and the Greater Good by Smith, J., Newman, K., Marsh, J., Keltner, D.

Gratitude is purposely the first step of the Hot Girl Walk, and after reading *The Gratitude Project*, you will understand how it's affected my life and the lives of so many others. This book is a collection of essays discussing the origins of gratitude, examples of gratitude throughout history, how it affects us on a neural level, and how we can use gratitude to better our lives and better humanity. It's a relatively new field of study but a highly relevant one. This book is a brilliant and hopeful perspective on the human race.

Glenn Fox, PhD, has been a great contributor in the science of gratitude and is a contributor on *The Gratitude Project*. He is a faculty member at the University of Southern California's Marshall School of Business. Fox received his PhD in Neuroscience from USC, where he focused on the neural correlation of gratitude, empathy, and neuroplasticity. He was also quoted in an article by the *Washington Post* saying:

"Those undertaking Hot Girl Walks may benefit from gratitude's virtuous cycle, beginning with exercising both one's mind and personal volition, reducing distraction, and focusing on personal abundance and strengths. The benefits of the Hot Girl Walk may be theoretically unlimited."

He has incredible insights and research on his website: https://glennrfox.com/.

Resources

Allen, Summer. *The Science of Gratitude*, May 2018. https://ggsc.berkeley.edu/images/uploads/GGSC-JTF_White_Paper-Gratitude-FINAL.pdf.

Clear, James. *Atomic Habits*. Avery, 2018.

Csikszentmihalyi, Mihaly. *Flow: The Psychology of Optimal Experience*. Harper Perennial Modern Classics, 2008.

Smith et al. *The Gratitude Project: How the Science of Thankfulness Can Rewire Our Brains for Resilience, Optimism, and the Greater Good*. New Harbinger Publications, 2020.

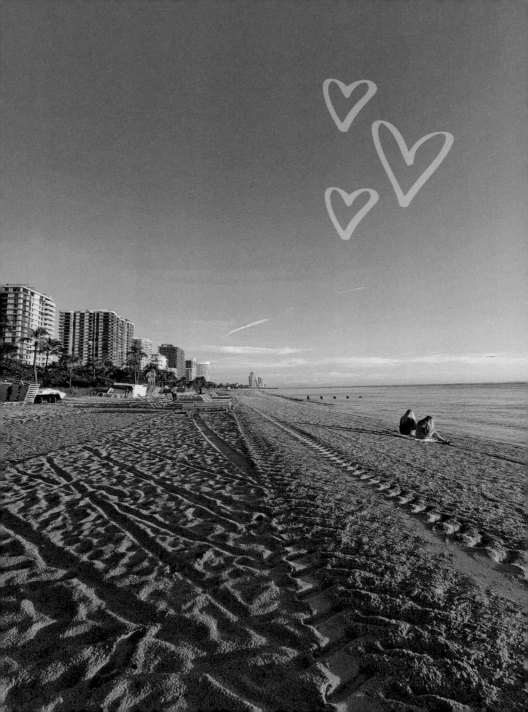

Acknowledgments

Writing this book has been (metaphorically) the longest Hot Girl Walk of my life. As a young girl, I never in a million years would have thought that I would be writing the Hot Girl manual. I grew up with doubts and a lack of confidence. It seemed like a sickness I could never quite shake. I spent the majority of my adolescence admiring confident women and seeing what I could do to replicate them. My original TikTok handle was @exactlyliketheothergirls (it has since changed) because I was tired of the narrative that we should work so hard to be different when there is so much to learn from each other. I am so honored to share these learnings with you.

Thank you to the Hot Girl Walk community. What I learn from this community is infinite. Every day I meet someone new who is uniquely incredible, and I feel honored to hear their stories. There is such strength in this sisterhood. I am humbled to be a part of your journeys. Keep Hot Girl Walk-ing.

I'd first like to thank Katey Abraham, my editor at Quarto, who helped make my thoughts make sense to the reader. These techniques and methods are ones I have only ever shared pieces of before, so putting them into words was challenging.

Many thanks to the person who saw the vision of this book and helped bring it to life, Rage Kindelsperger from Quarto. When Rage came to me with the idea for a book, it seemed like fate. Writing a book was a small seed in my mind, and I am so grateful that Rage helped me bring this to life.

Thank you to the Hot Girl Walk Ambassadors. You trusted me with this crazy vision of having Hot Girl Walks around the world, and you have helped me bring it to life in more ways than I could have imagined. You epitomize HOT in every way, and you are true leaders in the community. I am in awe of you every day!

Thank you to Catherine Hoffman and Jennifer Ko Craft, my lawyers who showed me the importance of protecting my intellectual property. You are both so incredible and have taught me what poise looks like in the face of chaos. You have been so supportive, both on and off the sidewalk, and have been mentors to me. I am honored to have you on my team.

Thank you to my friends and family for the constant support. Amber, who sits on FaceTime with me for hours and who has *literally* Hot Girl Walk-ed into a storm with me. My boyfriend Bryce, who is always holding the camera, cheering me on, and is my solace for when my inner critic comes out. Thank you to my brother, who has a gift for writing and seems to always find the right words. To my sister (and roommate during this process), who always finds the humor in everything, doesn't let me take myself too seriously, is definitely the creative one, and, last but not least, *my best friend!*

I'd next like to thank my dad, who has helped me see things through a positive light and find opportunity in life. We used to always say my dad lives life "on the rainbow" because of his relentless positivity, especially when things seem to be going wrong. Much of the time, it's still lost on me where the positivity comes from, but he's given me a valuable mindset when it comes to having a positive outlook on life. Additionally, my dad has always been a businessman giving me mini lessons on starting and growing a business. Starting Hot Girl Walk has been a culmination of the Dad MBA program. Starting a business called Hot Girl Walk may have been odd for my dad who is admittedly not the most in tune with social media or pop culture, but he always believes in me and has become Hot Girl Walk's biggest fan. You can usually catch him wearing a "STAFF" shirt at any Hot Girl Walk event.

Lastly, my mom has been the biggest inspiration for me. She was always the one to tell me about the power we have as women and has been the image of an inspiring woman. Growing up, she'd tell me tales of her life in corporate America in NYC, and I was honored to follow in her footsteps by going into sales after college. My mom was the very first person to tell me she'd support me in filing for a trademark and that my silly little TikToks had the power to inspire millions. She is my number one supporter, who encouraged me to leave the stability of my corporate job to pursue Hot Girl Walk full-time. My mom and I have worked hand-in-hand on Hot Girl Walk, and I could not be more grateful to have someone so strong in my corner. If you've had the chance to meet her, you know she is the QUEEN of confidence with her strong New York accent and fearlessness. I aspire to be like her, and I am immeasurably grateful for her support of me, not just in my business but throughout my life.

And thank you to everyone who has believed in me through this process and beyond. You're never Hot Girl Walk-ing through life alone.

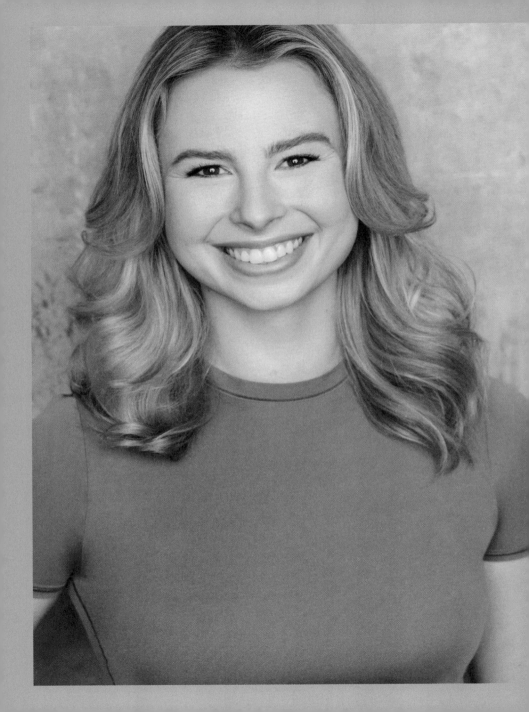

About *the* Author

Mia Lind is the creator and founder of the Hot Girl Walk and has been featured on CBS News, NBC News, *Vogue*, *Cosmopolitan*, the *New York Times*, *HuffPost*, and more. In 2020, she created the Hot Girl Walk to combine her passion of physical fitness with female- and self-empowerment. Hot Girl Walk events continue to spread across the world and have been hosted in some of the world's most populous cities, including Miami, New York, Boston, Los Angeles, Las Vegas, and London, as well as the Gold Coast, Australia so far.

Where to Find the Hot Girl Walk Community

Stay up-to-date on all things Hot Girl Walk to get more lessons and tips from Mia and the Hot Girl Walk community! Sign up on hotgirlwalk.com.

Everything you need to know about the Hot Girl Walk community can be found on Instagram @hotgirlwalk or at the website hotgirlwalk.com. Monthly community Hot Girl Walks are hosted in Los Angeles, Miami, New York City, London, and more. Follow to stay up to date on where to Hot Girl Walk.

First published in 2025 by Rock Point, an imprint of The Quarto Group,
142 West 36th Street, 4th Floor, New York, NY 10018, USA
(212) 779-4972 www.Quarto.com

EEA Representation, WTS Tax d.o.o.,
Žanova ulica 3, 4000 Kranj, Slovenia.
www.wts-tax.si

Rock Point titles are also available at discount for retail, wholesale, promotional, and bulk purchase.
For details, contact the Special Sales Manager by email at specialsales@quarto.com or by mail at
The Quarto Group, Attn: Special Sales Manager, 100 Cummings Center Suite 265D, Beverly, MA
01915 USA.

10 9 8 7 6 5 4 3 2 1

ISBN: 978-1-57715-549-2

Digital edition published in 2025
eISBN: 978-0-76039-858-6

Audiobook published in 2025
ISBN: 978-1-57715-5-584

Library of Congress Control Number: 2025935945

Group Publisher: Rage Kindelsperger
Editorial Director: Erin Canning
Creative Director: Laura Drew
Managing Editor: Cara Donaldson
Editor: Katelynn Abraham
Cover Design: Laura Drew
Interior Design: Casey Schuurman
Additional Photography: Mia Lind and Cole Nelson, pages 2 and 9
Author Photo: Stephanie Girard, page 158

Printed in Huizhou, Guangdong, China TT062025

This book provides general information on various widely known and widely accepted images
that tend to evoke feelings of strength and confidence. However, it should not be relied upon
as recommending or promoting any specific diagnosis or method of treatment for a particular
condition, and it is not intended as a substitute for medical or mental health advice or for direct
diagnosis and treatment of a medical or mental health condition by a qualified physician. Readers
who have questions about a particular condition, possible treatments for that condition, or possible
reactions from the condition or its treatment should consult a physician or other qualified health
care professional.